Analytical Procedures in Animal Nutrition and Feed Technology

Analytical Procedures in Animal Nutrition and Feed Technology

Authors

Vinod Kumar

Associate Professor, Department of Animal Nutrition, College of Veterinary Science and Animal Husbandry, U.P. Pt. Deen Dayal Upadhyaya Pashu Chikitsa Vigyan Vishwavidyalaya Evam Go-Anusandhan Sansthan (DUVASU), Mathura-281 001 (UP), Email: vinodsidhu@rediffmail.com, vinodsidhu@gmail.com, Contact: +91 9837636535

Muneendra Kumar

Assistant Professor, Department of Animal Nutrition, College of Veterinary Science and Animal Husbandry, U.P. Pt. Deen Dayal Upadhyaya Pashu Chikitsa Vigyan Vishwavidyalaya Evam Go-Anusandhan Sansthan (DUVASU), Mathura – 281 001 (UP), Email: muneendra82@gmail.com Contact: +91 9045546435

Raju Kushwaha

Assistant Professor, Department of Animal Nutrition, College of Veterinary Science and Animal Husbandry, U.P. Pt. Deen Dayal Upadhyaya Pashu Chikitsa Vigyan Vishwavidyalaya Evam Go-Anusandhan Sansthan (DUVASU), Mathura – 281 001 (UP), Email: rajuvet15@gmail.com Contact: +91 8791881240

SSPH

SATISH SERIAL PUBLISHING HOUSE

403, Express Tower, Commercial Complex
Azadpur, Delhi-110033 (India)
Phone : 011-27672852, Fax : 91-11-27672046
e-mail : info@satishserial.com, hkjain1975@yahoo.com
Website : www.satishserial.com

Published by :

SATISH SERIAL PUBLISHING HOUSE
403, Express Tower, Commercial Complex, Azadpur, Delhi-110033 (INDIA)
Phone : 011-27672852 Fax : 91-11-27672046
E-mail : info@satishserial.com, hkjain1975@yahoo.com

ISBN 978-93-86200-59-4

Composed, Designed & Printed in India

About the Authors

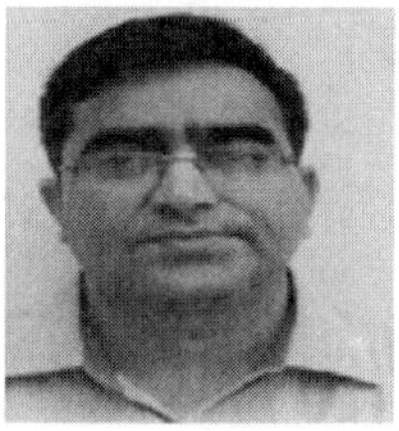

Dr. Vinod Kumar was born in village Pawti in Hapur district of Uttar Pradesh on 3th July 1976. He completed his graduation in Veterinary Science and Animal Husbandry (B.V.Sc. & A.H.) in 2001 from G.B. Pant University of Agriculture & Technology, Pantnagar, Uttrakhand. He completed his M.V.Sc. (Animal Nutrition) from IVRI, Izatnagar, Uttar Pradesh, in 2003 and Ph.D. (Animal Nutrition) from NDRI, Karnal, Haryana in year 2009. He started his carrier as Assistant Professor in 2007 in the Animal Nutrition division, F.V.Sc. & A.H., SKUAST-Jammu and subsequently at the Animal Nutrition department College of Veterinary Science and Animal Husbandry, DUVASU, Mathura from January, 2009. In June 2014, Dr. Kumar selected as Associate Professor in the same department. Since 2010, he is the officer Incharge of Department of Animal Nutrition. His work on the practical aspects of animal nutrition received considerable acclaim especially on mineral nutrition and unconventional feed sources. He involved himself in conducting research in area of trace element research, non conventional feed resources, and precision nutrition. He has guided four M.V.Sc and two Ph.D students. He formulated area specific mineral mixture (DUMIN-AS) for Braj region. He is lifetime member of Animal Nutrition Society of India, Animal Nutrition Association, Indian, Academy of Veterinary Nutrition and Animal Welfare, Indian Poultry Science Association and Indian Science Congress Association. Dr. Kumar has been executive committee member of Animal Nutrition Society of India and IPSA, India. He has published about 30 research articles in international and national journals, 5 laboratory manuals and contributed 3 chapters in books, delivered invited lectures and lead papers in various seminar/trainings/workshop etc. Dr Kumar has many prestigious award in various seminar and symposia like best paper presentation as oral and poster. He was recently given research excellence award by ETT-CRS. Dr Kumar is involved in various project of national importance like gokul gram mission and experiential learning.

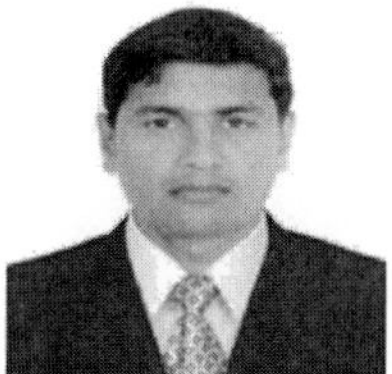

Dr. Muneendra Kumar born in village Bhawan Khera, Hardoi district of Uttar Pradesh on 5th July, 1982 did his B.V.Sc. & A.H. in 2007 from U.P. Pandit Deen Dayal Upadhyaya Pashu Chikitsa Vigyan Vishwavidyalaya Evam Go-Anusandhan Sansthan (DUVASU), Mathura. He qualified ICAR- Junior Research Fellowship for Masters degree programme and completed his M.V.Sc.

(Animal Nutrition) from ICAR-NDRI, Karnal, Haryana in 2009. Dr. Kumar awarded Institutional Fellowship and pursued his doctoral programme (Animal Nutrition) in the same institution. He became Assistant Professor in Department of Animal Nutrition on 19th October, 2011 at College of Veterinary Science, DUVASU, Mathura. Dr. Kumar had a deep involvement in teaching, research and extension on various facets of animal nutrition. His work on the micronutrient nutrition received considerable acclaim. Dr. Kumar awarded the prestigious VLIR-UOS Scholarship in 2014 for International Training Programme in Animal Nutrition organized by Gent University, Belgium. Dr. Kumar was recipient of K. Pradhan and VIFRA Young Scientist Award (2015) and many awards in category of oral and poster presentation. He is lifetime member of Animal Nutrition Society of India, Animal Nutrition Association, Indian Academy of Veterinary Nutrition and Animal Welfare, Society for Conservation of Domestic Animal Biodiversity, Indian Poultry Science Association, International Society for Environmental Information Sciences, The Indian Science Congress Association, Associated member of the be-troplive, the Belgian Platform on Tropical Animal Health and Production. He is executive (CEC) member of Animal Nutrition Society of India and Animal Nutrition Association. Dr. Kumar attended two international conferences at Belgium and several national conferences. He has published 13 research articles in international journals, 25 research articles in national journals, 4 laboratory manuals and contributed 2 chapters in books.

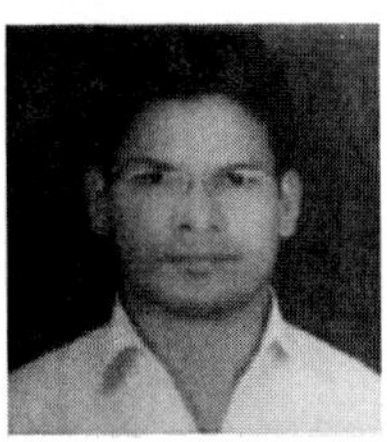

Dr Raju Kushwaha born on September 15, 1979 in Kanpur Nagar of U.P. graduated in Veterinary Science and Animal Husbandry from DUVASU, Mathura (2007). Dr. Kushwaha qualified ICAR- Junior Research Fellowship for Masters degree programme and completed his M.V.Sc. (Animal Nutrition) from ICAR-NDRI, Karnal, Haryana in 2009. He joined as Assistant Professor in Department of Animal Nutrition, College of Veterinary Science and Animal Husbandry, DUVASU, Mathura (U.P.) in June, 2014. Dr. Kushwaha involved in teaching, research and extension activities regarding to animal nutrition. He involved himself in conducting research in area of antinutritional factors. He is lifetime member of Animal Nutrition Society of India, Animal Nutrition Association and The Indian Science Congress Association. He has published 11 research articles and 2 laboratory manuals.

OFFICE OF THE DEAN
College of Veterinary Science & Animal Husbandry
U. P. Pt. Deen Dayal Upadhyaya Pashu Chikitsa
Vigyan Vishwavidyalaya
Evam Go Anusandhan Sansthan, Mathura. 281001

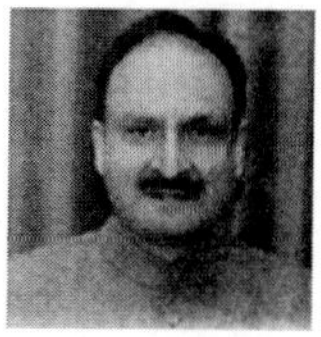

Prof (Dr.) Satish K. Garg
M.V.Sc. Ph. D., FNAVSc,
FNADSc, FST, SISVPT
DEAN

Date: October 31, 2017

FOREWORD

I am very glad to know that Drs. Vinod Kumar, Muneendra Kumar and Raju Kushwaha have authored the book titled "Analytical Procedures in Animal Nutrition and Feed Technology" keeping in view the requirements of students, scientists, teachers and others involved in the field of animal nutrition. This book will be very useful in understanding the basic principles and methodologies involved in preparation of different standard solutions, proximate analysis, fiber-fraction determination, estimation of minerals, vitamins, fatty acids and amino acids etc.

This book has been designed to give rapid and easy access to the recent and well-validated tests and techniques used in evaluation of feedstuffs, rumen fermentation studies including methane estimation, detection of adulterants, harmful constituents, and determination of pesticides residues in feedstuffs and animal products.

I am sure this book will enhance the practical knowledge and analytical skills of students, scientists and technicians involved in academics especially those who are involved in quality control in the feed-industry.

I heartily congratulate all the authors of this book and wish all success in their future endeavors and academic pursuits.

(Satish K. Garg)

Preface

Every sector of the livestock industry, the associated services and the wellbeing of both animals and humans are influenced by animal feeding. Proper animal feeding is the supply of a diet balanced in all nutrients and free from deleterious components. The availability of accurate, reliable and reproducible analytical data regarding nutrients composition is imperative for proper feed formulation. Also only reliable data can lead to the generation of sound scientific data. Therefore, better understanding of analytical procedures and laboratory techniques used in animal nutrition is required. The text in book represents an attempt to summarize and consolidate a considerable amount of information relative to principles, methodology and experimental techniques that are commonly used in animal nutrition studies. Basically, the text is an outline of the author's laboratory manuals with attempts made to expand and reference where possible. This book is designed to give rapid and easy access to the recent test and techniques used. The content can be divided into various sections including preparation of standard solution, proximate analysis, mineral and vitamin estimation, analysis of energy content, fatty acid and amino acid, enteric methane measurement, rumen liquor analysis, determination of quality of silage, detection of adulterants and harmful constituents in animal feedstuffs. The authors hopes that this book will also serve as useful reference to understand recent techniques like atomic absorption spectrometry, inductively coupled plasma-atomic emission spectrophotometer, gas and liquid chromatography, thin layer chromatography, high performance liquid chromatography and near-infrared-spectroscopy etc. Each section of book provides a structured approach to learning by covering the topics in a uniform and systematic format. The methods and techniques are detailed in a straight forward and lucid manner. This book will be useful for research students, teachers, scientists and laboratory analysts involved in feed analysis and quality control.

Our thanks to Dr. Debashis Roy, Dr. Shalini Vaswani and Dr. Avinash Kumar for the important contribution made in the preparation of this book. I appreciate the contribution of staff of animal nutrition department for providing us conducive environment for designing of this superior manuscript.

Authors

List of Tables

1.1 Molecular weight and equivalent weight of commonly used chemicals 5

1.2 Common examples of acid-base indicators 5

1.3 Amount of acid/alkali required for preparation of standard solution 9

2.1 Amount of biological sample taken for bio-chemical analysis 18

5.1 Classification of minerals 40

5.2 Elements detectable by atomic absorption spectrophotometer 46

6.1 Wavelengths used in the application of NIR-spectroscopy 55

6.2 NIR-wavelengths and their association with chemical structures 55

6.3 Error in NIR-spectroscopy 56

12.1 Composition of different solutions 94

12.2 Composition of rumen inoculum 95

13.1 Physical characteristics of rumen fluid 100

13.2 Chemical characteristics of rumen fluid 101

13.3 Microscopic examination of rumen protozoa 102

15.1 Confirmation of feeds by physical evaluation 120

15.2 Precise characteristics on microscopic identification 122

15.3 Visual examination of soybean meal when treated with urea-phenol red solution 127

15.4 Visual examination of presence of heavy metals in animal feed 129

16.1 Common anti-nutritional factors present in animal feeds and fodders 132

List of Figures

7.1 Diagram of bomb calorimeter 60
12.1 Components of permeation device 91
12.2 PVC collector canister (yoke) parts 91

Contents

About the Authors .... *v*
Foreword .... *vii*
Preface .... *ix*
List of Tables .... *xi*
List of Figures .... *xiii*

1. Preparation and Expression of Standard Solution 1
2. Preparation and Processing of Sample 11
3. Proximate Analysis 21
4. Estimation of Fibre Fraction 33
5. Determination of Mineral Content 39
6. Determination of Chemical Composition by Near-Infrared Spectroscopy 53
7. Determination of Energy Content 59
8. Fatty Acid Analysis 63
9. Amino Acid Analysis 67
10. Vitamin Analysis 71
11. Biological Methods for Feed and Fodder Evaluation 79
12. Enteric Methane Measurement in Ruminants 89
13. Rumen Liquor Analysis 97
14. Assessment of Nutritional Quality of Silage 113

15. Detection of Adulterants in Animal Feed 119

16. Detection of Anti-Nutritional Factors in Feed 131

17. Determination of Pesticide Residues 161

References 165

Appendices

Appendix-I: List of abbreviations 169

Appendix-II: Nutrient composition of common feedstuffs 172

Units and conversion 174

Frequently used standards of concentration 176

1

Preparation and Expression of Standard Solution

1.1. Standard solution 1

1.2. Expressing concentration of standard solution 1

1.3. Dilution 4

1.4. Indicator 5

1.5. Acid-base titration 6

1.6. Preparation of standard solution commonly used in nutritional analysis 6

1.1. Standard solution

A solution of known concentration is called the standard solution. A primary standard is a reagent that is extremely pure and stable; it not a hydrate/it has no water of hydration, and it has a high molecular weight. A secondary standard is a standard that is prepared in the laboratory for a specific analysis. It is usually standardized against a primary standard. The term secondary standard can also be applied to a substance whose active agent contents have been found by comparison against a primary standard.

1.2. Expressing concentration of standard solution

The concentration of a solution can be expressed in the following ways.

i) Molarity (M)

It is defined as the number of gram moles of solute dissolved in one litre of the solution.

$$\text{Molarity(M)} = \frac{\text{Number of gram moles of the solute}}{\text{Volume of the solution (litre)}}$$

Molarity of concentrated reagents

$$\text{Molarity(M)} = \frac{\text{Specific gravity (g / l)} \times \text{percentage (\%)} \times 1000}{\text{Mol. wt. (g / mol.)}}$$

ii) Molality (m)

Molality is defined as the number of moles of the solute dissolved in one kg of the solvent.

$$\text{Molarity(M)} = \frac{\text{Number of moles of the solute}}{\text{Mass of the solvent (kg)}}$$

iii) Normality (N)

It is defined as the number of gram equivalent of solute dissolved in one litre of the solution.

$$\text{Normality (N)} = \frac{\text{Number of gram equivalent of the solute}}{\text{Volume of the solution (litre)}}$$

Normality of concentrated reagents

$$\text{Normality (N)} = \frac{\text{Specific gravity (g / l)} \times \text{percentage (\%)} \times 1000}{\text{Eq. wt. (g / eq.)}}$$

iv) Relationship between molarity and normality

$$\text{Normality (N)} = \frac{\text{Weight (g)}}{\text{Equivalent weight (g / Eq.)}} \times \frac{100}{\text{Volume (ml)}}$$

$$\text{Molarity (M)} = \frac{\text{Weight (g)}}{\text{Molecular weight (g/ mol)}} \times \frac{100}{\text{Volume (ml)}}$$

$$\text{Equi va lent weight (Eq.wt.)} = \frac{\text{Molecular Weight (Mol.wt.)}}{\text{Normality (N)}}$$

Equivalent weight of acid is the molecular weight of acid/basicity of acid. Equivalent weight of base is the molecular weight of base/acidity of acid and equivalent weight of salt is the molecular weight of salt/charge present on ionic form. Molecular weight is the sum of atomic weight.

Weight, volume and weight-to-volume ratios

Weight percent (% w/w), volume percent (% v/v) and weight-to-volume percent (% w/v) express concentration as units of solute per 100 units of solution. Parts per million (ppm) and parts per billion (ppb) are mass ratios of grams of solute to one million or one billion grams of sample, respectively.

i) Weight by weight percentage (% w/w)

$$\% \, w/w = \frac{\text{g of solute}}{\text{100 g of solution}} = \frac{\text{g of solute}}{\text{g of solution}} \times 100$$

ii) Volume by volume percentage (% v/v)

$$\% \, v/v = \frac{\text{ml of solute}}{\text{100 ml of solution}} = \frac{\text{ml of solute}}{\text{ml of solution}} \times 100$$

iii) Weight by volume percentage (% w/v)

$$\% \, w/v = \frac{\text{g of solute}}{\text{100 ml of solution}} = \frac{\text{g of solute}}{\text{ml of solution}} \times 100$$

iv) Parts per million (ppm)

$$\text{ppm}(w/w) = \frac{\text{mg of solute}}{\text{kg of solution}} = \frac{\mu\text{g of solute}}{\text{g of solution}} = \frac{\text{ng of solute}}{\text{mg of solution}}$$

$$\text{ppm}(w/v) = \frac{\text{mg of solute}}{\text{litre of solution}} = \frac{\mu\text{g of solute}}{\text{ml of solution}} = \frac{\text{ng of solute}}{\mu\text{g of solution}}$$

v) Parts per billion (ppb)

$$\text{ppb}(w/w) = \frac{\mu\text{g of solute}}{\text{kg of solution}} = \frac{\text{ng of solute}}{\text{g of solution}} = \frac{\text{pg of solute}}{\text{mg of solution}}$$

$$\text{ppb}(w/v) = \frac{\mu\text{g of solute}}{\text{litre of solution}} = \frac{\text{ng of solute}}{\text{ml of solution}} = \frac{\text{pg of solute}}{\mu\text{g of solution}}$$

vi) Relationship between ppm and molarity and normality

$$\text{ppm} = \text{M} \times \text{Mol.wt.} \times 1000$$

$$\text{ppm} = \text{N} \times \text{Eq.wt.} \times 1000$$

vii) Mole fraction (X)

The mole fraction, X, of a component in a solution is the ratio of the number of moles of that component to the total number of moles of all components in the solution.

The mole fraction of A (X_A), in a solution consisting of A, B, C ... is calculated using the equation:

$$X_A = \frac{\text{Moles of A}}{\text{Moles of A + moles of B + moles of C + ...}}$$

To calculate the mole fraction of B (X_B), use

$$X_B = \frac{\text{Moles of B}}{\text{Moles of A + moles of B + moles of C + ...}}$$

1.3. Dilution

Whenever you need to go from a more concentrated (stock) solution to a less concentrated one, you add solvent to "dilute" the solution.

$$C1\,V1 = C2\,V2$$

Where, C1 is the concentration of the stock, V1 is the volume of the stock, C2 is the concentration of the final solution and V2 is the volume of the final solution.

$$N1\,V1 = N2\,V2$$

$$M1\,V1 = M2\,V2$$

Where, N1 is the normality of the stock solution, V1 is the volume of the stock, N2 is the required normality of the final solution and V2 is the required volume of the final solution. M1 is the molarity of the stock solution and M2 is the required molarity of the final solution.

Table 1.1. Molecular weight and equivalent weight of commonly used chemicals

S.No.	Chemical name	Formula	Mol. wt. (g/mol)	Eq. wt. (g/mol)
1.	Hydrochloric acid	HCl	36.5	36.5
2.	Sulfuric acid	H_2SO_4	98	49
3.	Nitric acid	HNO_3	63	63
4.	Potassium hydroxide	KOH	56	56
5.	Acetic acid	CH_3COOH	60	60
6.	Sodium hydroxide	$NaOH$	40	40
7.	Calcium hydroxide	$Ca(OH)_2$	74	37
8.	Ammonium hydroxide	NH_4OH	35	35
9.	Potassium dichromate	$K_2Cr_2O_7$	294	49
10.	Sodium thiosulphate	$Na_2S_2O_3 .5H_2O$	248	248
11.	Potassium permagnate	$KMnO_4$	158	31.6
12.	Sodium chloride	$NaCl$	58.5	58.5
13.	Potassium chloride	KCl	74.5	74.5

1.4. Indicator

An indicator is a chemical substance that undergoes a colour change at the endpoint. The endpoint of an acid-base titration can be determined using acid-base indicators. Acid base indicators are either weak organic acids or weak organic bases. The colour change of an indicator depends on the pH of the medium. The un-ionized form of an indicator has one colour, but its ionized form has a different colour.

Table 1.2. Common examples of acid-base indicators

S.No.	Indicators	pH range	Colour	
			Acid	Base
1.	Phenolphthalein	8.0 - 10.0	Colourless	Pink
2.	Methyl orange	3.1 - 4.4	Red	Orange
3.	Methyl red	4.4 - 6.2	Red	Yellow
4.	Phenol red	6.4 - 8.0	Yellow	Red
5.	Thymol blue	1.2 - 2.8	Red	Yellow
6.	Thymol blue	8.0 - 9.6	Yellow	Blue
7.	Methyl yellow	2.9 - 4.0	Red	Yellow

1.5. Acid-base titration

It is a method used to determine the strength of an acid or alkali and this type of titration is based on the neutralization reaction.

AH (acid) + BOH (base) = AB (salt) + H_2O (water)

Acid-base titration can be classified into the following types.

i) Strong acid-strong base titration: In this type, a strong acid is titrated against a strong base. Both the acid and base are of equal strength, so at the endpoint, the pH will be neutral. The indicators used are phenolphthalein and methyl orange.

ii) Strong acid-weak base titration: In this type, strong acid reacts with a weak base to form an acidic solution. So the pH of the solution is less than 7. Methyl orange is the indicator used to determine the endpoint.

iii) Strong base-weak acid titration: Here a strong base reacts with a weak acid to form a basic solution. So the pH of the solution is more than 7. In this type phenolphthalein is a suitable indicator for the determination of the end point.

iv) Weak acid-weak base titration: This type of titration is not very practical. Here both the acid and base are very weak so they do not ionize completely. So, it is difficult to determine the pH range around the end point and it is difficult to choose a suitable indicator for this type of titration.

1.6. Preparation of standard solution commonly used in nutritional analysis

i) Preparation of N/10 H_2SO_4

Equivalent weight of H_2SO_4 = 49 g, specific gravity = 1.84 g/ml and purity = 98%.

So, 26.63 ml of H_2SO_4 contain 49 g H_2SO_4. Actual amount of concentrated H_2SO_4 required for 1.0 litre of 1N H_2SO_4 = (100/98) × 26.63 = 27.17 ml. Thus, for 1.0 litre of N/10 H_2SO_4 solution, 2.72 ml of concentrated H_2SO_4 is required.

Procedure

Take 2.72 ml sulphuric acid in a beaker half-filled with distilled water. Transfer the contents and washings to a volumetric flask (1 litre capacity) and make volume up to the mark. Shake well and titrate this solution with 10 ml of N/10 Na_2CO_3 using mixed / methyl orange as an indicator. Repeat the titration to get at least three concordant readings.

Standardization

Suppose 10 ml of N/10 Na_2CO_3 = 9.5 ml of H_2SO_4

V1 N1 = V2 N2

10 x N/10 = 9.5 x N = 0.10526

To prepare 1 litre N/10 H_2SO_4, the volume of 0.10526 N acid required.

1000 x 0.1/0.10526 = 950 ml.

Take 950 ml of 0.10526 N acid and dilute it to 1 litre. Check it again with N/10 Na_2CO_3 for three times. It must neutralize equal volume of N/10 Na_2CO_3 solution. Label it as N/10 H_2SO_4.

ii) Preparation of N/10 NaOH solution

Molecular weight of NaOH = 40 g, acidity (number of replaceable OH group) = 1, equivalent weight of NaOH = 40, Therefore, 4 g of NaOH dissolved in 1 litre of solution will give N/10 NaOH solution.

Procedure

Weigh quickly 4 g NaOH in a beaker (as it is hygroscopic) and dissolve it in distilled water (preferably CO_2 free). Transfer the contents and the washings to a volumetric flask (1 litre capacity). Cool and then make volume up to the mark with distilled water. Shake well and standardize this solution against N/10 oxalic acid using phenolphthalein as an indicator. Label it as N/10 NaOH solution.

iii) Preparation of N/10 $KMnO_4$ solution

Molecular weight of $KMnO_4$ = 158 g. equivalent weight of $KMnO_4$ = 31.6 (the Mn in $KMnO_4$ exists in +7 state. In acidic medium, This Mn^{+7} goes to Mn^{+2} state and hence there is a net gain of 5 electrons. Therefore, the equivalent weight = 158/5 = 31.6 g).

Procedure

Dissolve 3.16 g of $KMnO_4$ in 1 litre of distilled water. Boil it for 10 to 15 minutes and then allow standing for few days and then filtering it through glass wool. Take 10 ml of N/10 oxalic acid in a beaker. Add 5 ml dilute sulphuric acid, warm it to 60 to 70°C and titrate against $KMnO_4$ from the burette till a light pinkish colour appears. Take three concordant readings.

Suppose 10 ml N/10 oxalic acid = 9.75 ml of $KMnO_4$

V1 N1 = V2 N2

10 x 0.1 N = 9.75 x N2

N2 = 0.10256

To prepare 1000 ml N/10 $KMnO_4$ solution, volume of $KMnO_4$ will be taken.

= (100 × 9.75 × 0.1)/ (10 × 0.1)

Now take 975 ml of prepared $KMnO_4$ solution and make it 1000 ml by adding distilled water.

Note: Ordinary or even pure distilled water contains traces of organic matter which reduces the $KMnO_4$ solutions. That is why the solution is boiled and kept for some time before standardization. In the absence of sufficient amount of dilute H_2SO_4 or due to the rapid addition of $KMnO_4$ in titration flask, brown turbidity (manganous oxide) may appear.

iv) Preparation of N/10 Na_2CO_3 solution

Molecular weight of Na_2CO_3 = 106, acidity of Na_2CO_3= 2, equivalent weight of Na_2CO_3 = 106/2 = 53. So 5.3 g Na_2CO_3 is required for each litre of solution to make N/10 Na_2CO_3. Na_2CO_3 is hygroscopic; therefore, it must be made perfectly anhydrous before it is weighed out.

Procedure

Take 6 to 7 g of Na_2CO_3 in a nickel crucible and heat it in a hot air oven at about 100°C for few hours so as to drive out any moisture and to convert any moisture preformed $NaHCO_3$ to Na_2CO_3. Cool in a desiccator and weigh exactly 5.3 g dried salt and dissolve it in a 5 to 10 ml freshly boiled distilled water. Transfer it to 1 litre measuring flask and make volume up to the mark with distilled water. Shake well and label it as N/10 Na_2CO_3 solution.

vi) Preparation of N/10 oxalic acid

Molecular weight of oxalic acid $(COOH)_2.2H_2O$ = 126 g, equivalent weight of = 63. 6.3 g is to be dissolved in 1 litre of distilled water to get N/10 oxalic acid solution.

Procedure

Weigh accurately 6.3 g oxalic acid and transfer it to a 1 litre volumetric flask, half-filled with distilled water. Shake well and make the volume up to the mark with distilled water. Label it as N/10 oxalic acid solution. If anhydrous oxalic acid (COOH) is available then dissolve 4.5 g of the acid in one litre of distilled water to get N/10 oxalic acid solution.

Table 1.3. Amount of acid/alkali required for preparation of standard solution

Normality	NaOH (g/L) (100% pure)	HCl (ml/L) (36% pure, 1.19 g/ml specific gravity)	H_2SO_4 (ml/L) (98% pure, 1.84 g/ml specific gravity)	HNO_3 (ml/L) (68% pure, 1.42 g/ml specific gravity)
0.1 N	4.0	8.5	2.7	6.5
0.5 N	20.0	42.6	13.6	32.6
1.0 N	40.0	85.2	27.2	65.2
1.5 N	60.0	127.8	40.8	97.8
2.0 N	80.0	170.4	54.3	130.4
2.5 N	100.0	213.0	67.9	163.0
5.0 N	200.0	426.0	135.9	326.0
10.0 N	421.0	853.0	271.7	652.0

□□□

2

Preparation and Processing of Sample

2.1. Sampling of concentrate 11

2.2. Sampling of roughage 12

2.3. Sampling during trial or experiment 13

2.4. Processing and preservation of samples 19

In animal nutrition experiment different kinds of substances like feed, fodder, silage, faeces, urine, milk, blood/plasma/serum etc. are processed for analyzing their chemical and biochemical characteristics. Following precautions should be taken during collection and processing of different kind of samples.

2.1. Sampling of concentrate

It includes sampling of individual concentrate ingredients and processed feed like compound cattle feed, pelleted feed, feed wafers, feed crumbles etc. This is a very important step in feed industry where raw feed ingredients like grains, cakes, agro-industrial byproducts and finished product are analyzed for their chemical constituents and therefore the price of those ingredients are determined. Parkhi (a tubular metallic probe having pointed end) is used for taking samples from bags. For sampling from bulk, a deep bin probe or thermo sampler is used.

i) Sampling from bags

It is impossible to take sample from each of the bag containing raw material coming to feed factory. So, a minimum number is set for sampling from bag. Bags are selected at random for sampling. Samples are taken out from the bags with the help of parkhi. All the samples are pooled together and a representative sample is taken for analysis.

Number of bag in the lot	Minimum number of bags to be sampled
Upto 30 bags	All bags
31 to 300 bags	30 bags
301 to 500 bags	30 bags + 10% excess

ii) Sampling from bulk

Feed ingredients are generally stacked in godowns. For sampling of feed ingredients from bulk sampler is inserted upto a desired depth into different places of bulk called spots. Number of spots depends upon the quantity of ingredient stored.

Bulk quantity	Number of spots for sampling
Upto 30 tones	30 spots
31 to 100 tones	50 spots
101 to 300 tones	50 spots+ 10% extra

After that all the spot samples are mixed and a representative sample is prepared. Representative sample is again divided into three sets. Each set contains three polythene bags containing at least 150g of representative sample. One set is kept with the buyer, second set is going to the seller and third one is kept at a mutually agreed place. These last set used if some dispute occurs between two parties.

2.2. Sampling of roughage

Roughage may be of different type and size (long and chaffed). In case of long fodder like hay (except legume hay), grass, un-chaffed straw or stover, the sample can be drawn by hand from different parts of stacks. For small stack of about 100 quintals, there should be 1 meter distance between two spots. If the stack is of 10 to 100 tones, the distance can be of 4 to 5 meters. For chaffed dry fodder like wheat straw the sampling can be done by a large inverted scoop with a long handle so that the scoop can be inserted upto a certain depth. The primary samples of long fodder are chaffed and mixed thoroughly. Three sets of secondary sample are packed into three bags of 1.5 kg each.

2.3. Sampling during trial or experiment

1. Sampling of feedstuffs

For precise estimation of chemical composition of feedstuff given to animal, sampling of each feed component is required. During digestion/metabolic trial, chemical composition of both offered and residual feedstuff, faeces and urine should be estimated. In case of lactating animals, milk samples are also collected.

i) Concentrate sample is taken after mixing the whole sample thoroughly. 100 g of sample is kept in a polythene bag and closed properly.

ii) Green fodder samples should be collected just before feeding to the animals. The fodder is chaffed thoroughly and about 200 to 300 g sample is taken in polythene packet. The packet should be closed immediately and DM content of the sample is measured as early as possible to avoid any error due to evaporation.

iii) After mixing the chaffed dry roughage thoroughly 100 g sample is taken in a polythene sheet. 50 g sample is taken for DM analysis and rest 50 g is kept in numbered polythene bag.

iv) Silage is cut into small pieces of 3 to 5 cm with hand chopper. After that it is mixed thoroughly and 500 g of sample is taken in a polythene bag. The bag is closed immediately to avoid moisture loss. A part of fresh sample is used for DM, ammonia nitrogen and volatile fatty acid analysis. Remaining sample is kept for other analysis.

2. Sampling of feed residue

Feed residue or ort or refusal is the left over feed by the animal after a day's (24 hrs) feeding. The left over is mixed thoroughly and about 200 gm of sample is taken in a polythene bag and closed immediately.

3. Sampling of faeces

Total faecal matter is collected for 24 hrs in a plastic or metal container. The collection should be done just after voiding of faeces. Mixed collected faeces thoroughly and a representative sample is taken in a polythene bag (see Table 2.1). In some species of animal like camel, sheep, goat, rabbit and deer, the faeces is in the form of pellets. The pellets should be broken down properly before mixing the whole faeces. DM content of the sample is estimated as early as possible to avoid any error due to evaporation. Dried sample is kept for further analysis. For estimating nitrogen content of faeces, a particular amount (depends on total faeces voided) of faeces is collected in a wide mouth container and 5ml of 25% of H_2SO_4 is added.

4. Sampling of urine

Whole urine is collected for a day in a plastic container. 25 ml of diluted H_2SO_4 (1:4) should be kept in that container before starting the collection to prevent the loss of volatile nitrogen content of urine. Total urine excreted for 24 hrs is mixed thoroughly and sample is taken in a plastic bottle and closed properly (see Table 2.1).

5. Sampling of milk

Take milk sample from lactating animals in a plastic container of 100 ml capacity (see Table 2.1). Add 2 to 3 drops of potassium dichromate or mercuric chloride (as a preservative) and keep bottle in deep freeze at – 20 °C for further analysis.

6. Blood collection

A. In cattle

Blood can be collected from the jugular vein in cattle of all ages or from the tail (coccygeal) vein of older cattle. A variety of collection devices vacuutainer, bleeding tubes, syringe and needle may be used. Restraint should ensure quick, easy and safe collection of the sample causing minimal distress.

a) Procedure for jugular venipuncture using vacuutainer needle and tubes :

   i) Before sample collection, ensure that the animal is effectively and humanely restrained to avoid injury to the animal and/ or study personnel.

   ii) Disinfect venipuncture area with alcohol.

   iii) Occlude the vein by applying digital pressure in the jugular groove located in the lower neck.

iv) Place a vacuutainer needle attached to a vacuutainer holder into the distended jugular vein at a 45° angle cranial to the jugular groove.

v) Once needle is positioned in the vein, insert a vacuutainer into the needle to collect the blood.

vi) When the desired volume has been collected (5 ml minimum suggested) remove the occluding pressure from the vein.

vii) Detach the tube from the needle and withdraw the needle from the jugular vein.

viii) You can collect more than 1 tube by repeating steps 7 and 8.

ix) Label the vacuutainer tubes with the sample ID.

b) Procedure for jugular venipuncture using syringe and needle

I. Jugular bleeding

i) Restrain cow with the head elevated and the jugular groove exposed.

ii) Raise the jugular vein by placing pressure at the base of the jugular groove.

iii) Pass the needle through the skin and into the vein by a firm thrust directed at an angle of 20° to the skin surface.

iv) Withdraw the blood sample.

II. Tail bleeding (coccygeal venipuncture)

i) Restraint should prevent the cow from moving away during the procedure.

ii) Raise the tail vertically with one hand until it is horizontal with the ground.

iii) Approximately 150 mm from the base of the tail, locate the groove lying in the ventral midline of the tail.

iv) Midway along the body of a coccygeal vertebra, insert the needle perpendicularly to the surface of the skin to a depth of a few millimeters.

v) Withdraw blood sample.

vi) Apply pressure to the venipuncture site after withdrawal of the needle until the bleeding stops.

B. In sheep and goats

Blood should be collected from the jugular vein. The procedures for blood collection are identical to those described for cattle, with the exception of the possibility of shearing the bleeding area on the neck for easier viewing of the vein. The sheep/goat's head should be turned opposite to the side of collection, once again at a 30° angle. Restraint of the head is accomplished by using the elbow and the upper arm to keep it held off to the side. This leaves both hands available for the blood collection. The easiest way to locate the vein is to draw an imaginary line from the middle of the sheep/goat's eye down the side of the neck. The vein can be located by applying pressure with the thumb or fingers in the groove on either side of the trachea. The pressure will cause the vein to pop up and be easy to feel or see if the area has been shaved. Proceed as with cattle, using a vacuutainer collection system or syringe and needle.

C. In swine

Blood can be collected from the external jugular vein, or the cranial vena cava, using a 1", 20G needle and a 5cc syringe. This technique requires the head to be restrained and elevated parallel to the ground, typically using a snout snare. In pigs weighing less than 50 kg, blood can be collected further caudally (and more medially) in the jugular groove, nearer the manubrium from anastomose of internal and external jugular vein. For pigs weighing less than 20 kg, a technician will manually restrain the pig on his lap, holding the forelegs in one hand, and the animal's head in the other. Then a maximum of 5.0 to 10 ml may be collected from the jugular vein. The marginal ear veins are the only veins that are easily visible on pigs of any size. Usually there are three prominent veins. The lateral or central vein is usually the largest of these. These veins may also be punctured for blood collection. An alternative venipuncture site is the caudal auricular (marginal ear) vein, though this typically yields low blood volumes (< 1 ml). A small needle (22 G or 23 G) should be used for this vein.

D. In camel

Blood can be collected from the jugular vein in camels of all ages, though it is recommended that this be undertaken on animals while they are in sternal recumbency (kush position), well restrained, or sedated. The lateral thoracic vein or caudal epigastric i.e. milk vein may be used but should only be targeted in animals where physical or chemical restraint prevents kicking.

a) Procedure for jugular venipuncture using vacuutainer needle and tubes :

   i) Before blood collection, ensure that the animal is effectively and humanely restrained to avoid injury to the animal and/or study personnel.

   ii) Disinfect venipuncture area with alcohol.

   iii) Occlude the vein by applying digital pressure in the jugular groove located in the lower neck. Alternatively, a rolled towel affixed with a rope over the withers can be applied at the same level to act as a temporary incomplete tourniquet.

   iv) Place a vacuutainer needle, attached to a vacuutainer holder, into the distended jugular vein at a 45° angle cranial to the jugular groove.

   v) Once the needle is positioned in the vein, insert a vacuutainer into the needle and collect the blood.

   vi) When the desired volume has been collected (5 ml minimum suggested), remove the occluding pressure and detach the tube from the needle.

   vii) Detach the needle from the jugular vein and apply pressure to the venipuncture site after withdrawal of the needle until the bleeding stops.

   viii) If more than one tube of blood is required, repeat steps 7 through 9 with occluding pressure.

   ix) Label the vacuutainer tubes with sample ID.

   x) If vacuutainer needles are unavailable, a 5 cc syringe and 18 G or 19 G needle can be used. Invert each tube several times to mix.

b) Procedure for jugular venipuncture using syringe and needle

   I. Jugular bleeding

      i) Restrain camel with the head elevated and the jugular groove exposed.

ii) Disinfect venipuncture area with alcohol.

iii) Raise the jugular vein by pressure at the base of the jugular groove.

iv) Pass the needle through the skin and into the vein by a firm thrust directed an angle of 20° to the skin surface.

v) Withdraw blood sample.

vi) Apply pressure to the venipuncture site after withdrawal of the needle until the bleeding stops.

II. Lateral thoracic/caudal epigastric vein bleeding

i) Restraint should prevent the camel from moving away or kicking during the procedure.

ii) Identify the lateral thoracic vein, caudal to the point of the elbow's olecranon process.

iii) Pass the needle through the skin and into the vein by a firm thrust directed an angle of 20° to the skin surface.

iv) Withdraw blood sample.

v) Apply pressure to the venipuncture site after withdrawal of the needle until the bleeding stops.

Table 2.1. Amount of biological sample taken for bio-chemical analysis

S.No.	Animal	Sample amount			
		Faeces (parts of total faeces)	Urine (ml)	Milk (ml)	Blood (ml)
1	Adult cattle	1/200	100	50	8-10
2	Adult buffalo	1/200	100	50	8-10
3	Adult goat	1/50	100	50	3-5
4	Adult sheep	1/50	100	50	3-5
5	Adult camel	1/200	100	50	8-10
6	Adult pig	1/50	100	50	3-5
7	Calf	1/50	100	-	3-5
8	Kid	1/10	100	-	2-3
9	Lamb	1/10	100	-	2-3
10	Poultry	50 g		-	2-2.5

Note: Water sampling is required during metabolism trial. Take 50 to 100 ml of drinking water in a plastic or glass container of 150 ml capacity.

2.4. Processing and preservation of sample

Samples required processing and preservation because it takes some time for analysis after collection. 100 g of representative sample of feedstuffs, residues and faeces is dried at hot air oven at 100±1°C and grind in a laboratory mill to pass a 1 mm sieve. The ground sample is kept in air tight polythene bag for further analysis of chemical composition. A level is pasted over the bag detain about sample number, kind of study and date of sampling. For gross energy estimation sample is dried at 60±1°C in hot air oven. Wet faeces sample is mixed with a known volume H_2SO_4 (25% v/v) and kept in a wide mouth bottle with proper closing for further analysis of nitrogen. A know amount of urine aliquot is stored in a Kjeldahl flask after proper numbering for nitrogen estimation. For gross energy estimation, 5 ml of urine sample is collected in stoppered glass or polythene tube and 2 to 3 drops of mercuric chloride is added as preservative. Fat in milk is estimated by Gerber's method on the day of collection. For other estimation milk is preserved adding 2 to 3 drops of potassium dichromate or mercuric chloride and kept in deep freeze.

❑❑❑

3

Proximate Analysis

3.1. Determination of moisture or dry matter content 22

3.2. Determination of total ash content 23

3.3. Determination of acid insoluble ash content 24

3.4. Determination of crude protein content 25

3.5. Determination of crude fat or ether extract content 27

3.6. Determination of crude fibre content 28

3.7. Determination of nitrogen free extract content................ 30

3.8. Limitation of proximate analysis 30

The proximate analysis is a scheme for routine description of animal feedstuffs devised in 1865 by Wilhelm Henneberg and Friedrich Stohmann of the Weende Experiment Station at the University of Gottingen, Germany. It is often referred to as the Weende's System of Analysis. Under the scheme various nutrients that have some common properties are grouped together and analyzed. Proximate analysis allows us to make legitimate comparisons of feeds on the basis of specific nutrients. The system consists of determinations of following six components:

1. Moisture/dry matter (DM)
2. Ash
3. Crude fat (ether extract; EE)
4. Crude protein (CP)
5. Crude fibre (CF)
6. Nitrogen free extract (NFE)

3.1. Determination of moisture or dry matter content

Dry matter (DM) or, more specifically, moisture determination is probably the most frequently performed analysis in the nutrition laboratory. It is an important analysis, in that the concentration of other nutrients is usually expressed on a DM basis (as a percentage of the DM). It gives information about the characteristics of the feed, whether it is succulent or dry feed stuff. It also gives the information about suitability of storage of feedstuff. The feed stuffs containing more than 15% of moisture are not safe to be stored in bulk as there will be growth of fungus and mould. Fermentation may also take place which lead to combustion. Determination of water content in feed is important since the relative cost of feed per unit of nutritional value is also calculated on DM basis. For preservation of fodder as silage, determination of water is essential since best silage can only be prepared when the water content in the fodder is between 60 - 65%. Common methods of DM analysis are as follows:

S.No.	Method	Occasion for use
1.	Oven drying	Most mixed feed, feeds and fodders, hay and range grasses with 85-99% DM
2.	Freeze drying	High moisture and fermented feed
3.	Saponification	High moisture and fermented feed
4.	Vacuum drying	Meat or tissue samples

When feed sample is subjected to the temperature of 100 ± 5°C till the constant weight is attained, all the moisture present in the feed gets evaporated.

Procedure

i) Chop or grind the sample received in the laboratory to particular size.

ii) Dry aluminum tray or cup in oven at 100 °C for 15 to 30 minutes. Cool in a dessicator, weigh and record its empty weight.

iii) Weigh accurately about 50 to 100 g of air dried samples in aluminum tray or 5 to 10 g in aluminum cup and record its weight.

iv) Place the tray or cup with sample in hot air oven maintained at 100 ± 5 °C and dry for 6 to 8 hrs.

v) Cool in a desiccator and weigh.

vi) Repeat the process of heating, cooling and weighing until the difference between two successive weighing is less than 1 mg.

Precaution

i) In some feeds having high decomposition matter like sugars, higher temperature is not desired; hence, the range of temperature should be 70 to 80 °C for 2 hrs.

ii) Special arrangements are done to estimate the moisture content of the samples like silages containing volatile fatty acids, otherwise there might be over estimation of moisture.

iii) For the samples which are liquid or pasty in nature (molasses), estimation of moisture is done by modified method.

iv) The samples which are classified as tubers have to be chopped down in thin slices and without any loss of time it should be transferred into hot air oven.

v) Time required for drying ranges from 6 to 24 hrs according to the nature of sample. It is very necessary to observe the temperature range of 100 ± 5 °C. Since the excess of temperature will remove not only moisture but also destroy other nutrients.

Calculation

$$\text{Moisture}(\%) = \frac{W1 - W2}{W1 - W2} \times 100$$

Where, W is the empty weight of tray or cup (g), W1 is the weight of tray or cup with sample (g) and W2 is the weight of tray or cup with sample after drying (g).

$$\text{DM}(\%) = 100 - \text{moisture percent in the sample}$$

3.2. Determination of total ash content

When a feed sample is subjected to high temperature (600 ± 30 °C), the organic part gets burnt leaving only inorganic part which is called as total ash. The part of ash which is soluble contains all mineral elements and high content of insoluble ash indicates poor quality of feed because it represents sand and silica. Total ash content is negatively correlated with energy content of feed.

Procedure

i) Find out the weight of a clean dry silica crucible/basin.

ii) Place about 2 g of sample and weigh this to find out accurate weight of the sample taken.

iii) Carefully place the weighed crucible over electric burner. The crucible should be partially opened.

iv) The sample will get charred with initial expulsion of smoke.

v) Place the crucible in a muffle furnace and heat to 600 ± 30 °C for 2 hrs. At this temperature all organic matter will be burnt leaving behind inorganic content.

vi) Remove the crucible from the furnace carefully and cool it in a dessicator to room temperature and weigh again.

Calculation

$$\text{Total ash content (\%)} = \frac{W3 - W1}{W2 - W1} \times 100$$

Where, W1 is the weight of empty silica crucible (g), W2 is the weight of silica crucible with sample (g) and W3 is the weight of silica crucible and ash after complete ashing (g).

What is obtained after complete combustion of a sample is total ash. It comprises of two portions: The portion that is soluble in dilute acids (acid soluble ash) contains all essential minerals and that is the useful portion of the ash. Other portion, insoluble in dilute acids (acid insoluble ash; AIA) consists of mainly sand and silica. For the most part, AIA represents impurity or adulteration.

3.3. Determination of acid insoluble ash content

That portion of the total ash which is insoluble in dilute HCl is called AIA. It contains sand and silica, which has no physiological role to play in animal body. Plant materials like straw, husk, stem and stalks are highly lignified or woody and are rich in silica. Sand may also find entry into feeds due to faulty handling in the field or used as an adulterant.

Procedure

i) Prepare the total ash (see 3.2).

ii) To the silica basin containing total ash add 40 ml of 1:4 HCl. Keep silica basin on hot plate (at low temperature) for digestion.

iii) After the digestion, the color of content of the silica basin will change to yellow.

iv) Cool the silica basin and filter the contents through the Whatman filter paper 42 in volumetric flask.

v) Wash the silica basin several times with hot distilled water till it becomes acid free.

vi) Test the filtrate drops at the tip of the funnel with blue litmus paper. After making it acid free make the volume to 250 ml in a volumetric flask by adding cold distilled water.

vii) Label it with necessary details and use aliquot of acid soluble ash for mineral analysis.

viii) Return the filter paper residues to the silica basin and keep it in the hot air oven at 135 °C for 1 hr.

ix) After complete drying char the filter paper at flame.

x) Ignite it in a muffle furnace at 600 ± 30 °C for 2 hrs.

xi) After complete ashing remove the silica basin, put it in desiccator. Cool it to room temperature and weigh it.

Calculation

$$\text{AIA}\,(\%\,\text{DM basis}) = \frac{100\,(\text{W2} - \text{W})}{\text{W1} - \text{W}}$$

Where, W is the weight of the silica basin (g), W1 is the weight of silica basin with dried material (g) and W2 is the weight of silica basin with the AIA.

3.4. Determination of crude protein content

The protein content is estimated on the assumption that all the nitrogen in the feed exists in the form of protein. As the protein contains 16% nitrogen, the value for CP is obtained by multiplying the nitrogen content by the protein factor (100/ 16 = 6.25). The nitrogen compounds in the sample are converted to ammonium sulphate by acid digestion with concentrated boiling sulphuric acid. The acid digest is cooled and diluted with distilled water and steam distilled with a strong alkali (sodium hydroxide). The released ammonia is condensed into a boric acid mixed indicator. The ammonia in the boric acid is quantified by titration with standard sulphuric acid.

Procedure

i) Weigh around 2 g of dried feed sample and transfer it into Kjeldahl flask.

ii) Add 10 g of the digestion mixture (copper sulphate: sodium sulphate or potassium sulphate: 1: 10) and 20 ml of concentrated sulphuric acid.

iii) Place flask on a digestion rack, turn the heater on and regulate the temperature (415 °C).

iv) When the charred material is dissolved and digest turns clear bluish green colour, boil for 1 hr.

v) Allow flask to cool and then gently add distilled water to makeup volume.

vi) Add 10 to 20 ml of 50% sodium hydroxide to the diluted digest in the Kjeldahl flask.

vii) Steam distill the mixture and collect 125 ml of distillate in a 25 ml boric acid mixed indicator (13.3 mg of methyl red in 10 ml of distilled alcohol and 6.66 mg of methylene blue in 50 ml of distilled water prepared separately, both mixed together in one litre volumetric flask and the volume made up to the mark using 4% boric acid solution) taken in an Erlenmeyer flask.

viii) Titrate contents of the Erlenmeyer flask with 0.143 N Sulphuric acid solution.

Calculation

$$CP(\%) = \frac{\text{Titre value} \times \text{Volume made out of digested sample} \times 0.002 \times 6.25 \times 100}{\text{Volume of aliquot taken} \times \text{Weight of the sample}}$$

$$CP(\%\,DM\ \text{basis}) = \frac{\%\,CP \times 100}{\%\,DM\ \text{of the sample}}$$

Where, 0.002 is the nitrogen equivalent of standard sulphuric acid (0.143 N sulphuric acid = 0.002g or 2 mg). The equivalent is derived from equation $2NH_3 + H_2SO_4 = (NH_4)_2SO_4$. In the equation, 2 units of nitrogen is reacting with 1 unit of sulphuric acid = (14 x 2) 28 units of nitrogen is reacting with 98 units of sulphuric acid. Therefore, 7 units of sulphuric acid can react with 2 units of nitrogen or 7 mg (contained in 1 ml of N/7 Standard sulphuric acid) of sulphuric acid is equivalent to 2 mg of nitrogen.

3.5. Determination of crude fat or ether extract content

The ether extract (EE) is that fraction of feedstuff which is obtained when the feedstuff is subjected to continuous extraction with petroleum ether. This includes besides the fats, cholesterol, free fatty acids, lecithin, chlorophyll, resins, volatile oils and plant sterols. These substances other than crude fats are termed as pseudo-fat. Since the proportion of the components of the EE will be variable. In composition in different foods, the energy supply from the EE in the oil cakes would be mostly the fats but in the green fodders large proportion of chlorophyll, volatile oils, carotenoids, etc. would also be there. The EE content is variable in various feeds and fodders. The EE is determined by Soxhlet ether extraction apparatus (consists of condenser at the top, Soxhlet or extractor siphon in the middle and receiver flask at the bottom.

Procedure

i) Set the Soxhlet apparatus in position.

ii) Take thimble and find out its weight.

iii) Transfer about 3 to 5 g of sample into the thimble and find out the correct weight of the sample by weighing the thimble with the sample.

iv) Plug the mouth of the thimble with cotton wool, to avoid the escape of material from the thimble during extraction.

v) Slide the thimble with the contents into the Soxhlet extractor and fix the lower end of the Soxhlet extractor to the oil flask underneath. Then fix the condenser above the Soxhlet extractor.

vi) Adjust the water circulation for efficient and uniform cooling of the condensing unit.

vii) The Soxhlet apparatus is placed over an electrical heater/ hot plate.

viii) From the top end of the apparatus pour about 100 ml of petroleum ether (B.P. 40-60°C) and plug the mouth with cotton.

ix) Run the extraction for 8 hrs till the collecting ether in the extractor is clean.

x) Dismantle the apparatus on the completion of extraction. Remove the extractor with the flask from the condenser. Remove the thimble with its contents. Place it in the oven for drying. When dried find out the weight of the thimble with the extracted residue.

xi) Remove the Soxhlet flask with the extract. Transfer it to a hot air oven (80 °C) for evaporating the petroleum ether for 1 hr, cool it in a desiccator and weigh.

Calculation

$$EE(\%) = \frac{W3 - W2}{W1 - W} \times 100$$

Where, W is the weight of empty thimble (g), W1 is the weight of thimble with sample (g), W2 is the weight of empty receiver flask (g) and W3 is the weight of receiver flask with EE (g).

3.6. Determination of crude fibre content

Crude fibre (CF) is that fraction of total carbohydrates which is not digested after successive boiling with dilute acid and dilute alkali. CF consists of cellulose, hemicellulose, pentosans and small fractions of lignin. The bulkiness of feed is correlated with the CF. CF absorbs moisture in the intestine and gives normal distention to digestive tract. This promotes the peristaltic movements of intestine which is helpful for voiding the digesta from the intestine. Roughages contain high proportion of CF and are indigestible part of ruminant ration. CF content of feed is negatively correlated with its nutritive value.

When moisture and fat free sample is boiled first with dilute acid (1.25 % H_2SO_4) and then with dilute alkali (1.25% NaOH) the soluble carbohydrates and protein go into solution and are extracted. The undissolved residue left behind represents cellulose; hemicellulose and lignin which put together are called as CF. When the residue after drying and weighing is heated at 600 °C, the fibre content is obtained by deducting the weight of ash from the weight of dried residue.

Procedure

i) Weigh 2 to 3 g of the sample on previously weighed glaze paper.

ii) Transfer the sample in 1000 ml capacity spoutless beaker with a mark made at 200 cc level with a glass pencil.

iii) See that the condensing flask fixes well over the beaker leaving no space. The condensing flask is filled with cold water. The purpose of keeping a condensing flask filled with cold water is for condensing back the evaporating acid to the beaker. This maintains the volume of the acid without any reduction.

iv) Add 200 ml of 1.25 % H_2SO_4 in the beaker containing sample and immediately connect a flask with reflux condenser and heat so that the contents begin to boil.

v) Continue the boiling for exactly 30 minutes. During boiling keep the volume constant. To avoid foaming add few drops of iso-amyl alcohol, if necessary.

vi) Filter the content of a beaker in a conical flask through muslin cloth (18 threads/cm^2) held over the glass funnel.

vii) Wash the residue on cloth with boiling water till residue gets acid free. Test with blue litmus paper.

viii) The acid digested residue is then subjected to alkali digestion. For this, transfer the acid digested material from muslin cloth back to the original beaker and pour 200 ml of 1.25 % NaOH into original beaker.

ix) Place over the heater and fix a condensing flask over this and heat to boil the content for 30 minutes.

x) After 30 minutes, remove the condenser; transfer the contents of the beaker to a filtering funnel. The residue is washed repeatedly with distilled water till it is alkali free. This is tested by catching one or two drops of the filtrate over red litmus. If it remains red it indicates that the residue is free from alkali.

xi) When the residue is free from alkali squeeze the cloth well to dry the residue. Transfer the residue, without any loss, to a clean silica crucible.

xii) The crucible is placed in preheated hot air oven (110 °C) over night. This is to drive off the moisture completely.

xiii) After complete drying, the crucible is cooled in desiccator. It is weighed along with the residue. Heat the crucible with electrical bunsen in order to ash the residue. Continue the heating till you obtain a whitish ash. Cool the crucible to room temperature and find out the weight.

Calculation

$$CF(\%) = \frac{W3 - W2}{W1 - W} \times 100$$

Where, W is the weight of glaze paper (g), W1 is the weight of glaze paper with sample (g), W2 is the weight of silica basin with ash residue (g) and W3 is the weight of silica basin with digested dried residue (g).

3.7. Determination of nitrogen free extract content

Nitrogen free extract (NFE) is a component of the proximate analysis but it is measured by difference rather than by analysis. NFE includes all the nutrients which are not assessed by the prior methods of proximate analysis and consists mainly of digestible carbohydrates, vitamins and other non-nitrogen soluble organic compounds. Since the result is obtained by subtracting the percentages calculated from each nutrient from 100, any errors in evaluation will be reflected in the final calculation of NFE as well.

$$NFE(\% \text{ as such basis}) = 100 - (CP\% + EE\% + CF\% + \text{Total Ash}\% + \text{Mositure}\%)$$

$$NFE(\% \text{ as DM basis}) = 100 - (CP\% + EE\% + CF\% + \text{Total Ash}\% + \text{Mositure}\%)$$

3.8. Limitation of proximate analysis

i) The proximate principles are not chemically and nutritionally pure but are the mixture of substances having common properties; hence it is termed as proximate principles.

ii) Proximate method results in under estimation of CF, since part of lignin and hemi cellulose gets dissolved during alkali digestion, which in turn leads to over estimation of NFE.

iii) NFE is calculated by difference; hence any experimental error may change the NFE value.

iv) In estimation of EE, along with true fats (triglycerides), the pseudo-fats also get estimated.

v) In protein estimation, along with true proteins, the NPN substances also get estimated, hence it is called CP.

vi) Minimum importance is given to micro-nutrients.

vii) The practical aspects like palatability and cost are not considered.

□□□

4

Estimation of Fibre Fraction

4.1. Determination of neutral detergent fibre content 33

4.2. Determination of acid detergent fibre content 35

4.3. Determination of acid detergent lignin content 36

4.4. Determination of acid detergent insoluble nitrogen content 37

4.5. Determination of total digestible nutrients........................ 38

P.J. Van Soest (1963) developed detergent method of determination of fibre fraction in feedstuffs to rectify the defects in proximate principles of estimating CF and NFE. Insoluble fibre fraction in feed is determined as neutral detergent fibre (NDF), acid detergent fibre (ADF) and acid detergent lignin (ADL). NDF fraction contains hemicelluloses, cellulose, lignins and is a general measurement of "total" fibre. The ADF content is an indication of the proportion of the cell wall framework substances cellulose, lignin and lignin-nitrogen compounds.

4.1. Determination of neutral detergent fibre content

Detergent method for estimation of fibre content in feedstuff provides more accurate values in comparison to proximate analysis. Neutral detergent fibre (NDF) divides the DM of feeds and fodders into completely soluble and insoluble materials. The insoluble material in neutral detergent solution (NDS) is cell wall contents (NDF). The cell contents are determined from the differences between percent cell wall and 100.

1. Neutral detergent solution

a) Sodium lauryl sulphate	30.00 g
b) Disodium ethylene diamino tetra acetate (EDTA) dehydrate	18.61 g
c) Sodium borate decahydrate	6.81 g
d) Disodium hydrogen phosphate	4.56 g
e) 2-ethoxy ethanol	10.00 ml
f) Distilled water	1.00 L

2. Decahydronaphthalin (Decalin)
3. Acetone

Procedure

i) Take 0.5 to 1.0 g air dry and ground sample into a beaker of refluxing apparatus.

ii) Add 100 ml NDS in the beaker. Reflux the content for 60 minutes from the onset of boiling.

iii) Filter the reagent in sintered glass crucible by using vacuum pump.

iv) Rinse crucibles with approximately 50 ml hot distilled water until all traces are removed.

v) Rinse with acetone repeatedly until drained liquid is cleared.

vi) Wash the beaker and filtrate thrice with hot distilled water followed by twice with acetone.

vii) Dry the crucible in hot air oven at 100 °C for overnight.

viii) Cool to room temperature in desiccator and weigh it.

Calculation

Calculate the NDF content as percent cell wall constituents and estimate cell soluble material by subtracting the value from 100.

$$\text{NDF content } (\%) = \frac{\text{Wo - Wt}}{\text{Ws}} \times 100$$

Where, Wo is the weight of cell wall constituents and crucible (g), Wt is the weight of oven dry empty glass crucible (g) and Ws is the weight of sample (g).

The ash residue left in the crucible after muffle furnace ashing at 550 °C for 3 hrs is reported as ash soluble in neutral detergent.

$$\text{NDF ash } (\%) = \frac{\text{Wa - Wt}}{\text{Ws}} \times 100$$

Where, Wa is the weight of crucible with ash (g), Wt is the weight of oven dry empty glass crucible (g) and Ws is the weight of sample (g).

$$\text{Cell content (\% as DM basis)} = 100 - \text{NDF (\% as DM basis)}$$

4.2. Determination of acid detergent fibre content

Acid detergent fibre (ADF) is highly indigestible part of forage and includes cellulose, lignin, silica and insoluble forms of nitrogen but not hemicellulose. Forages with higher ADF are lower in digestible energy than forages with lower ADF. ADF is the residue remaining after boiling a feed and forage samples in acid detergents solution (ADS). ADF is often used to calculate digestibility, total digestible nutrients (TDN) and net energy for lactation (NE_l). ADF determination is a preparation step for lignin determination.

Procedure

i) Take 0.5 to 1.0 g air dry and ground sample into a beaker.

ii) Add 100 ml ADS [contains 20 g cetyl trimethyl ammonium bromide (CTAB) in 1000 ml 1N H_2SO_4] and 2 ml decalin in the beaker.

iii) Heat to boiling for 5 to 10 minutes. Reduce the heat and reflux the content for 60 minutes from the onset of boiling.

iv) Filter through previously weighed sintered glass crucible by using vacuum pump.

v) Rinse crucibles with approximately 50 ml hot water until all traces are removed.

vi) Rinse with acetone repeatedly until drained liquid is cleared.

vii) Wash the beaker and filtrate thrice with hot distilled water followed by twice with acetone.

viii) Dry the crucible in hot air oven at 100 °C for overnight.

ix) Cool to room temperature in desiccator and weight crucible with sample.

x) Ash residues for 3 hrs at 550 °C. Cool to room temperature in desiccator. Weight crucibles with residues.

Calculation

$$\text{ADF content (\%)} = \frac{\text{Wo - Wt}}{\text{Ws}} \times 100$$

Where, Wo is the weight of crucible with ADF (g), Wt is the weight of oven dry empty glass crucible (g) and Ws is the weight of sample (g).

$$\text{ADF ash (\%)} = \frac{\text{Wa - Wt}}{\text{Ws}} \times 100$$

Where, Wa is the weight of crucible with ash (g), Wt is the weight of oven dry empty glass crucible (g) and Ws is the weight of sample (g).

4.3. Determination of acid detergent lignin content

Lignin is the indigestible non-carbohydrate component of forages. Acid detergent lignin (ADL) represents the indigestible NDF fraction. ADL is the percentage of plant material which is insoluble in 72% sulphuric acid. This analysis is performed sequentially on ADF residue. Treatment with 72% sulfuric acid dissolves cellulose. Ashing the residue will determine the crude lignin fraction including cutin. Permanganate lignin procedure separates cutin and lignin. Lignin reduces digestibility and has been used to predict digestibility.

Procedure

i) Prepare the ADF (see 4.2).

ii) Place the crucible on the glass tray by keeping one end of the tray 2 cm higher so that the acid can be drained away from the crucibles.

iii) Cover the content of the crucible with cooled (15 °C) 72% H_2SO_4 and stirred with a glass rod to break all lumps.

iv) Fill the crucible almost half with acid and stir. Let glass rod remain in the crucible. Refill the crucible with 72% H_2SO_4 and stir at hourly interval as the acid drained away. Crucible does not need to be kept full at all times. Three additions are sufficient.

v) Keep crucible overnight at 100 °C, cool in desiccator and weigh.

vi) Ignite the crucible in muffle furnace at 550 °C for 3 hrs. Cool in desiccator and weigh.

Calculation

$$\text{ADL content (\%)} = \frac{\text{Wa - Wo}}{\text{Ws}} \times 100$$

Where, Wa is the weight of crucible with residues left after acid treatment (g), Wo is the weight of crucible with ash (g) and Ws is the weight of sample (g).

4.4. Determination of acid detergent insoluble nitrogen content

Acid detergent insoluble nitrogen (ADIN) is a measure of the nitrogen remaining in the ADF residue of a feed sample. Acid detergent fibre crude protein (ADFCP) is ADIN expressed as crude protein on a dry matter basis. The percentage of ADIN on DM basis is determined from the total ADF residue that is trapped in filter paper.

Procedure

i) Dry filter paper overnight at 100 °C and weigh it.

ii) Weigh 1 g air dry sample in 600 ml capacity beaker.

iii) Add 100 ml ADS and boil content for 1 hr on refluxing apparatus.

iv) Filter onto filter paper using funnel with vacuum suction.

v) Wash beaker with hot distilled water to remove all fibre particles into filter paper.

vi) Use blanks (filter paper washed with ADF solution) to estimate nitrogen in paper and reagents.

vii) Soak twice with boiling water after filling funnel with vacuum off for 2 minutes.

viii) Rinse twice with acetone by filling funnel with vacuum off for 2 minutes before vacuum drying.

ix) Leave folded filter paper with residues in oven at 105 °C for 8 hrs or overnight.

x) Weigh hot filter paper with residues.

xi) Transfer paper residue into Kjeldahl digestion tube.

xii) Add additional 5 ml sulfuric acid to digest filter paper.

xiii) Determine nitrogen in residue by standard Kjeldahl.

xiv) Titrate with 0.01 N standard acid.

Calculation

$$\text{ADIN content } (\%) = \frac{(\%\text{N in Wt} - \%\text{ N in Wo})}{(\text{Ws} \times \%\text{DM})} \times 100$$

Where, N is the nitrogen content, Wo is the weight of dry filter paper (g), Wt is the weight of hot filter paper with residues (g) and Ws is the weight of air dry sample (g).

4.5. Determination of total digestible nutrients

Total digestible nutrients (TDN) represent energy based on a carbohydrate equivalent basis.

TDN is calculated as the digestible CP, CF, NFE and EE × 2.25 added together. The formula for calculating TDN% is as follows:

$$\text{TDN}(\%) = \text{DCP}\% + \text{DCF}\% + \text{DNFE}\% + (\text{DEE}\% \times 2.25)$$

The digestible fat (EE) is multiplied by the factor 2.25. This is the correction factor for arriving al digestible carbohydrate equivalent from digestible fat according to Atwater fuel values (carbohydrate: 4 Kcal/g; fat 9 Kcal/g) because the values have taken account of only digestible losses in case of these nutrients. TDN value of a feedstuff can be used to derive other form of energy by using the following relationship:

$$1\,\text{kg TDN} = 4.409\,\text{Mcal DE} = 3.616\,\text{Mcal ME}$$

❑❑❑

5

Determination of Mineral Content

5.1. General principle of mineral estimation 40

5.2. Preparation of acid soluble ash 41

5.3. Estimation of calcium by titration method 41

5.4. Estimation of phosphorus 43

5.5. Determination of mineral by atomic absorption spectrophotometer 45

5.6. Determination of mineral by inductively coupled plasmaatomic emission spectrophotometer 49

Minerals are required for tissue growth and the regulation of body functions. The classification of the essential minerals into major or macro elements and trace or micro or minor elements depends upon their concentration in the animal or amounts required in the diet. Normally major elements are present in the animal body in a concentration greater than 50 mg/kg and are required at more than 100 mg/kg diet. Whereas, trace elements are present in the animal body in a concentration lesser than 50 mg/kg and are required at less than 100 mg/kg diet.

Table 5.1. Classification of minerals

S.No.	Major elements	S.No.	Trace elements
1.	Calcium (Ca)	1.	Iron (Fe)
2.	Phosphorus (P)	2.	Zinc (Zn)
3.	Sodium (Na)	3.	Copper (Cu)
4.	Potassium (K)	4.	Molybdenum (Mo)
5.	Chlorine (Cl)	5.	Selenium (Se)
6.	Sulphur (S)	6.	Iodine (I)
7.	Magnesium (Mg)	7.	Manganese (Mn)
		8.	Cobalt (Co)
		9.	Chromium (Cr)

The essentiality of other elements like nickel (Ni), vanadium (V), tin (Sn), silicon (Si), fluorine (F), arsenic (As) listed as possible or newer elements by some authorities. But confirmation of essentiality is still lacking.

5.1. General principle of mineral estimation

Ash is the inorganic residue remaining after the water and organic matter have been removed by heating in the presence of oxidizing agents, which provides a measure of the total amount of minerals within a food. Analytical techniques for providing information about the total mineral content are based on the fact that the minerals can be distinguished from all the other components within a food in some measurable way. The method chosen for a particular mineral analysis depends on the reason for carrying out the analysis, the type of food analyzed and the equipment available. The major physicochemical characteristics of minerals that are used to distinguish them from the surrounding matrix are: their low volatility; their ability to react with specific chemical reagents to give measurable changes; and their unique electromagnetic spectra. The most effective means of determining the type and concentration of specific minerals in foods is to use atomic absorption or emission spectroscopy. Instruments based on this principle can be used to quantify the entire range of minerals in feed, fodder and animal body, often to concentrations as low as a few ppb/ ppm.

5.2. Preparation of acid soluble ash

i) Prepare the total ash (see 3.2).

ii) To the silica basin containing total ash add 40 ml of 1:4 HCl. Keep silica basin on hot plate (at low temperature) for digestion.

iii) After the digestion, the color of content of the silica basin will change to yellow.

iv) Cool the silica basin and filter the contents through the Whatman filter paper 42 in volumetric flask.

v) Wash the silica basin several times with hot distilled water till it becomes acid free.

vi) Test the filtrate drops at the tip of the funnel with blue litmus paper. After making it acid free make the volume to 250 ml in a volumetric flask by adding cold distilled water.

vii) Label it with necessary details and use aliquot of acid soluble ash for mineral analysis.

5.3. Estimation of calcium by titration method

When a solution containing calcium (Ca) is treated with saturated ammonium oxalate ($C_2H_8N_2O_4$), all the Ca present in sample is precipitated as calcium oxalate (CaC_2O_4). The precipitate, when treated with conc. H_2SO_4 gets dissolves forming calcium sulphate ($CaSO_4$) and liberating free oxalic acid ($C_2H_2O_4$) which is quantitatively estimated by titrating against N/10 $KMnO_4$ solution to arrive at the Ca content present in the given sample (Talpatra *et al.*, 1940).

Procedure

i) Pipette out an aliquot 10 ml from the stock ash solution into 250 ml beaker (see 5.2). Dilute it up to 100 ml by adding distilled water.

ii) To this add 10 ml saturated solution of ammonium oxalate and 2-3 drops of 0.2% alcoholic solution of methyl red indicator.

iii) Mix solution thoroughly with glass rod. The solution turns red as the ash has been extracted with HCl in the preparation of the acid soluble ash.

iv) The solution which is acidic in nature is neutralized by adding dilute 5% ammonium hydroxide solution drop by drop to just reach the pH range in the alkaline medium.

v) Boil the content of the beaker for 10 to 15 minutes and cool. This makes the precipitate of calcium oxalate granular.

vi) Wash the precipitate with hot distilled water and filter through Whatman filter paper 40 to make it chloride free.

vii) Test the filtrate with 1% silver nitrate ($AgNO_3$) solution to detect presence of chlorides. The real technique of filtration is keeping maximum quantity of calcium oxalate in the original beaker than pouring it on filter paper during filtration.

viii) Transfer the filter papers to original beaker in such a way that outer surface of filter paper sticks to inner wall of beaker. Then dissolve the precipitate with jet of distilled water. About 50 ml of distilled water may be used for this purpose.

ix) Add 10 ml of conc. H_2SO_4 to the original beaker. Care should be taken to avoid burning of filter paper. Place the filter paper in beaker in such a way that outer side of the filter paper sticks to inner wall of beaker.

x) Heat the beaker till the contents start boiling. During titration the temperature of the contents should not go below 80 °C.

xi) Titrate the solution (when it is hot) against N/10 $KMnO_4$ solution. The pink colour appearing after running $KMnO_4$ solution should remain at least for 15 seconds. Record the volume of N/10 $KMnO_4$ required for titration.

Calculation

$$\text{Ca (\%)} = \frac{\text{cc of N/10 KMnO4 required} \times 0.002 \times \text{A.F.}}{\text{Weight of sample}} \times 100$$

1 ml of N/10 KMnO4 = 0.002 g of Ca

Where A.F. is aliquot factor

$$\text{A.F.} = \frac{\text{Volume of aliquot prepared}}{\text{Volume of aliquot taken}}$$

Chemical Reactions

The calcium in 'soluble ash' is precipitated as calcium oxalate. This is then dissolved in dilute sulphuric acid.

$$Ca\,(COO)_2 + H_2SO_4 \rightarrow CaSO_4 + (COOH)_2$$

The calcium is determined volumetrically by titrating the solution with standard $KMnO_4$.

$$2KMnO_4 + 3H_2SO_4 + 5(COOH)_2 \rightarrow 2MnSO_4 + K_2SO_4 + 10CO_2 + 8H_2O$$

The reaction involved in titration with $KMnO_4$ is

$$5Ca(COO)_2 + 2KMnO_4 + 8H_2SO_4 \rightarrow 5CaSO_4 + 2MnSO_4 + K_2SO_4 + 10CO_2 + 8H_2O$$

5.4. Estimation of phosphorus

A. Volumetric method

In volumetric method, phosphorus is converted to phospho-ammonium-molybdate $[(NH_4)_3PMo_{12}O_{40}]$ by addition of diammonium molybdate $[(NH_4)_2MoO_4]$. The precipitate is then dissolved in excess of standard alkali. The quantity of alkali required to dissolve the precipitate is indirectly determine by back titrating with standard HCl or HNO_3.

Procedure

i) Take 10 ml from acid soluble aliquot in 250 ml beaker (see 5.2) and make volume 100 ml by adding distilled water.

ii) Take 10 ml of 20% ammonium molybdate (precipitant) in a test tube.

iii) Take 10 ml of conc. HNO_3 in another test tube.

iv) Pour both these reagents in a common stream in the beaker containing aliquot.

v) Stir the contents of beaker vigorously with glass rod till canary yellow colour precipitate is formed and allow the beaker to stand for overnight.

vi) Transfer the supernatant fluid to the Whatman filter paper 42 with the help of conical flask and funnel. As the filtration proceeds, continue transferring the supernatant liquid in small portions. When all the supernatant liquid is thus transferred to the funnel, wait for complete filtration. The next step is washing of the precipitate.

Washing of the precipitate

vii) Transfer 10 ml of 3% KNO_3 on the filter paper containing the precipitate. Mix well. Allow to settle.

viii) Transfer the supernatant fluid to the filtering funnel. Wait for complete filtration. By this time transfer another 10 ml of 3% KNO_3 to the beaker, mix well and allow it to settle.

ix) When the previous filtration is complete, transfer the supernatant fluid from the beaker to the beaker paper. (Don't start filtration unless the previous filtration is complete. Continue the washing and filtration till the filtrate is acid free.

x) Test the filtrate by taking blue litmus if litmus paper turns red. Precipitate is not acid free and further washing is needed.

Dissolving the precipitate

xi) When the filtrate is free from acid, gently take the filter paper and make it into a pulp. Now wash the sides of the beaker with distilled water. The entire content are now yellow.

xii) Add known amount of N/10 NaOH till the yellow colour disappears and the contents become colourless except for the white filter paper residues.

xiii) Stir well and add 1 to 2 drops of phenolphthalein indicator. Pink colour appears indicating excess of alkali.

Back titration

The amount of excess alkali added is found out by back titration with N/10 HCI or HNO_3. From the total amount of 0.1N NaOH added, the quantity of acid required for titration is deducted to arrive at the actual quantity of alkali required for dissolving the precipitate. The end point of titration is pink to colourless. Note the initial and final readings.

Calculation

$$P(\%) = \frac{0.0001347 \times N/10OH \text{ required} \times A.F.}{\text{Weight of feed sample}} \times 100$$

1 ml of N/10 NaOH = 0.0001347 g of P

Where A.F. is aliquot factor.

B. Spectrophotometric method

Procedure

i) Take 10 ml from acid soluble aliquot in 250 ml beaker (see 5.2) and make volume 100 ml by adding distilled water.

ii) Mix molybdovanadate reagent in 10 ml aliquot and dilute it to 50 ml in a volumetric flask.

iii) Standard P solutions also mixed with reagent.

iv) Take absorbance of unknown and standard solutions at 400 nm in a spectrophotometer.

Calculation

By using data from the standards, we can calculate the P concentration in the unknown sample by following ways.

i) Standard curve method: We can plot concentration vs. absorbance and extrapolate concentrations for unknown samples.

ii) Linear regression: We can calculate an equation for the line that we have "guessed at" in standard curve method by using simple linear regression. The form of the equation will be:

$$Y = b_o + b_1X$$

Where, Y is the predicted concentration, bo is the Y intercept, b_1 is the slope of the line, X is the absorbance of standards.

5.5. Determination of mineral by atomic absorption spectrophotometer

Flame atomic absorption spectrophotometry (FAAS) is a very common technique for detecting minerals in feeds, fodders and animals. The technique is based on the fact that ground state metals absorb light at specific wavelengths. Metal ions in a solution are converted to atomic state by means of a flame. Light of the appropriate wavelength is supplied and the amount of light absorbed can be measured against a standard curve. The element being analyzed is dissociated from its chemical bond and is placed in an un-ionized state. The amount of light absorbed is proportion to the amount of the element that is present which , in turn, is proportional to the amount of the element that is continuously fed into the flame. To transfer the analyte to free atoms, different types of atomizer are in use, the flame and the graphite furnace types being the most often used. Typical detection limits of FAAS are of the order of 1 to 100 μgL^{-1}. Graphite furnace atomic absorption spectrometry (GFAAS), offering detection limits which are about 20 to 200 times lower than for FAAS. The GFAAS and FAAS measurement principle is the same. The difference between these two techniques is the way the sample is introduced into the instrument. In GFAA analysis, an electrothermal graphite furnace is used instead. AAS is a well established technique for the quantification of nearly 50 elements in a variety of sample types with sensitivity at the ppm level or less.

Table 5.2. Elements detectable by atomic absorption spectrophotometer

S.No.	Elements	S.No.	Elements	S.No.	Elements
1	Sodium (Na)	18	Lithium (Li)	35	Palladium (Pd)
2	Magnesium (Mg)	19	Beryllium (Be)	36	Indium (In)
3	Potassium (K)	20	Scandium (Sc)	37	Tin (Sn)
4	Calcium (Ca)	21	Titanium	38	Antimony (Sb)
5	Chromium (Cr)	22	Vanadium (V)	39	Tellurium (Te)
6	Manganese (Mn)	23	Gallium (Ga)	40	Caesium (Cs)
7	Iron (Fe)	24	Germanium (Ge)	41	Barium (Ba)
8	Cobalt (Co)	25	Boron (B)	42	Tantalum (Ta)
9	Nickel (Ni)	26	Silicon (Si)	43	Tungsten (W)
10	Copper (Cu)	27	Rubidium (Rb)	44	Rhenium (Re)
11	Zinc (Zn)	28	Strontium (Sr)	45	Iridium (Ir)
12	Arsenic (As)	29	Yttrium (Y)	46	Platinum (Pt)
13	Selenium (Se)	30	Zirconium (Zr)	47	Gold (Au)
14	Aluminum (Al)	31	Niobium ((Nb)	48	Mercury (Hg)
15	Lead (Pb)	32	Mendelvium (Md)	49	Titanium (Ti)
16	Silver (Ag)	33	Ruthenium (Ru)	50	Bismuth (Bi)
17	Cadmium (Cd)	34	Rhodium (Rh)		

Procedure

The main steps in AAS measurements are: 1. sample preparation, 2. aspiration of sample into the flame/or graphite furnace, 3. conversion of the sample into free atoms and the gaseous atomic state (atomic cloud) formation, 4. absorption of the monochromatic radiation by the ground state atoms from the atomic cloud, 5. measurement of the transmitted radiation intensity and 6. extraction of the quantitative formation from the registered signal.

1. Sample preparation

The feed sample must be converted to liquid form prior to analysis. This is mostly done by dry ashing or wet digestion or by using microwave to digest the samples, leaving a solution that can then be analyzed.

Dry ashing: Preparation of acid soluble ash (see 5.2).

Wet ashing

i) Weigh 2 to 3 g of feed sample into a 600 ml Kjeldahl flask or 250 ml beaker.

ii) Add 25 ml conc. nitric acid (HNO_3) and boil gently for 50 minutes to oxidize al easily oxidizable matter.

iii) Cool the solution and add slowly 10 ml of 70 to 72% perchloric acid ($HClO_4$).

iv) Boil very gently, adjusting heater regulator as necessary, until solution is clear and dense white fumes appear.

v) Cool the solution slightly and add 50 ml de-ionized water and boil to drive out any remaining NO_2 fumes.

vi) Cool, dilute and filter through Whatman filter paper 1 and then dilute to specific volume and mix thoroughly.

Microwave digestion

Feed samples digested by dry or wet ashing method take more time and laborious, also. The most convenient and time saving method of sample preparation for the determination of minerals using AAS, inductively coupled plasma atomic emission spectroscopy (ICP-AES) or inductively coupled plasma mass spectrometry (ICP-MS) is by using microwave digestion system. To carry out the digestion in microwave oven, the following steps are to be performed:

i) Clean and dry the vessels before starting the digestion.

ii) Weigh 20-40 mg sample (maximum 100 mg) and add decomposition reagents [consisted of HNO_3 (65%), HCl (30%), H_2O_2 (30%), H_2SO_4 (97%), and $HClO_4$ (60%)].

iii) Insert the liner into the dry vessels jacket.

iv) Expand the seals and close the vessels and vessel Jacket.

v) Load the rotor and start the digestion.

vi) End the digestion, vent the pressure vessels and unload rotor.

2. Analysis of minerals

The following steps to be performed while working with AAS instrument:

i) Switch on the main switch, air compressor, instrument and exhaust hood.

ii) Open the fuel gas cylinder.

iii) Open the software, if any, attached with instrument.

iv) Select the method for desired mineral and give the sample information.

v) Set up the particular lamp for specific mineral and ignite the flame.

vi) Check the instrument sensitivity with characteristic concentration check value solution for desired mineral at a particular wavelength.

vii) Calibrate the instrument with standard and draw the standard curve.

viii) Run the unknown samples and calculate the concentration of minerals in unknown samples using sample weight, dilution factor, etc.

Calculation

$$\text{Mineral } (\mu g/g) = \frac{\text{Concentration of mineral in sample (mg/L)} \times \text{volume made(ml)}}{\text{Weight of sample (g)}}$$

Note: If further dilution is made from extract solution that can be multiplied as dilution factor. The standard solutions must be prepared to be nearly identical in composition with the samples as possible in order to minimize the errors. Ultra-pure reagents and solvents should be used.

5.6. Determination of mineral by inductively coupled plasma-atomic emission spectrophotometer

Inductively coupled plasma-atomic emission spectrometry (ICP-AES) presents distinct advantages when compared with other instrumental techniques used for mineral estimation, due to the wide coverage of determinable elements, the power of detection and the excellent precision and accuracy attainable with modern instruments of high resolution. In contrast to AAS (single element analysis at a time), the high energy ICP-AES allows the simultaneous recording of different spectral lines, which enables multi elements analysis in a single sample.

ICP-AES is a well-established technique for determining inorganic constitutes in various types of samples (especially animal origin). Basically, the sample solution is introduced into the excitation device as a fine spray, where the solvent evaporates leaving the dehydrated salt. The salt is dissociated into free gaseous atoms in the ground state and then a certain fraction of these atoms can be raised to an excited electronic state, by the effect of high temperature. These excited atoms return to their ground state emitting photons of characteristics wavelength. The intensity of the emitted radiation is proportional to the concentration of analyte in the sample. The main steps in ICP-AES measurement are: 1. conversion of sample to free atom gas, 2. excitation of the atoms and their ions to higher electronic states, 3. measurement of the emission wavelength and intensities and 4. extraction of quantitative and qualitative information from these signals.

1. Sample preparation

Sample preparation is same as described above under AAS method and procedure (see 5.5). In AAS, standard solution of a particular element is run at a time, while in ICP-AES, standard solution of multiple elements should be run at a time.

2. Analysis of minerals

i) Turn on computer, printer, and main power of the ICP-AES.

ii) Open valve on argon tank and confirm tank volume is 500 lbs; if argon tank volume is <500 lbs, change out tank before starting analyses. Verify that gas regulator on argon tank is set at 80 psi, if not adjust to 80 psi.

iii) Set up inlet and outlet tubing on peristaltic pump and turn the pump switch on to the low setting. Insert inlet tubing into blank; verify computer clockwise movement of fluid through tubing (inlet tube goes from sample to nebulizer and outlet tube goes from nebulizer to the collection vessel on the floor under the instrument); make sure tubing is not crimped or impeded anywhere along the pathway. Make sure the pump is continually drawing up liquid.

iv) Verify the nebulizer is set at the proper flow rate.

v) Ignite the plasma; allow the instrument to warm up to about 20 minutes to stabilize the wavelengths, then it will be ready to begin analysis.

vi) Retrieve prior developed method file from the operating software. Verify that the method file has all the elements of interest, the right wavelength for each element, and the concentrations of the calibration standards.

vii) Follow instructions to initiate running sample analysis in the order of blanks (Millipore water), standards, and unknown sample.

viii) Following completion of sample analysis, run 5% HNO_3 through the ICP for 5 minutes, followed by deionized water for 10 minutes.

ix) Turn off peristaltic pump; loosen the two screws and flip the lever back into the up position to release tension on the inlet and outlet tubes.

x) Turn off main power. Close valve on argon tank.

xi) On the computer, escape out of the ICP analysis programme; turn off computer and printer.

Calculation

Data generated by ICP-AES will either be the instrumental signals or the concentration or both. The concentrations reported are the concentration of the liquid digest sample in, for example, mg/L. This will need to be converted to µg/g dry weight for solid samples using the formula:

$$mg/kg = mg/L \times V/W$$

Where, V is the volume of digested solution (ml) and W is the dry sample weight (g).

❑❑❑

6

Determination of Chemical Composition by Near-infrared Spectroscopy

6.1. Principle of working of near infrared-spectroscopy 54

6.2. Instrumentation 54

6.3. Choice of wavelengths 55

6.4. Technical errors in near infrared-spectroscopy 56

6.5. Procedure 56

6.6 Precautions 57

6.7. Advantages of near infrared-spectroscopy 57

6.8. Limitations of near infrared-spectroscopy 58

Limitation with proximate analysis and other methods can be overcome by analyzing feed and fodder samples with near-infrared (NIR)-spectroscopy. NIR-spectroscopy is a spectroscopic method that uses the near-infrared region of the electromagnetic spectrum (700 nm to 2500 nm). Norris and his colleagues (1965) developed the first application of NIR spectroscopy to measure water in grains and seeds. The technology uses simple sample preparation methods (drying and grinding), is very rapid and inexpensive. It avoids the problems of organic and other chemical waste disposal, and there are few if any hazards associated with the technique because it uses no toxic or corrosive reagents. NIR-spectroscopy is widely applied in animal nutrition for determining the quality of forages, grains, and grain products, oilseeds, fats, and oils, dairy products, eggs, meat, and other products. It is widely used to quantify the composition of feeds and fodders because it meets the criteria of being accurate, reliable, rapid, non-destructive, and inexpensive.

6.1. Principle of working of near infrared-spectroscopy

NIR-spectroscopy works on the principle of Beer-Lambert law. The Beer-Lambert law describes the relationship between the concentration of a solute and the amount of light absorbed by the solution. When infrared radiation is incident on a solid sample, some of it is reflected from the surface of the sample. Another proportion of the radiation enters the sample and may be absorbed within it. Radiation which is not absorbed may be transmitted through the sample or reflected from it. While the Beer-Lambert law generally describes the relationship between radiation diffusely reflected from a solid sample and characteristics of that sample, the path length of diffusely reflected radiation cannot be predicted because it is scattered by random reflections, refractions and diffractions within the sample. The amount of radiation reflected from the sample is quantified as the reflectance (R) of the sample. There is an almost linear relationship between log (1/R) and the concentration of an absorbing component. The log (1/R) curve is comparable to an absorption curve with peak values occurring at wavelengths which correspond to absorption bands in the sample.

6.2. Instrumentation

Instrumentation for NIR- spectroscopy is similar to instruments for the UV-visible and mid-infra red ranges. There is a source, a detector, and a dispersive element (such as a prism, or, more commonly, a diffraction grating) to allow the intensity at different wavelengths to be recorded. Fourier transform NIR- spectroscopy instruments using an interferometer are also common, especially for wavelengths above 1000 nm. Depending on the sample, the spectrum can be measured in either reflection or transmission. Common incandescent or quartz halogen light bulbs are most often used as broadband sources of NIR radiation for analytical applications. Light-emitting diodes are also used; they offer greater lifetime and spectral stability and reduced power requirements. For high precision spectroscopy, wavelength-scanned lasers and frequency combs have recently become powerful sources, albeit with sometimes longer acquisition timescales. When lasers are used, a single detector without any dispersive elements might be sufficient. The type of detector used depends primarily on the range of wavelengths to be measured. Silicon-based charge-coupled devices (CCDs) are suitable for the shorter end of the NIR range, but are not sufficiently sensitive over most of the range (over 1000 nm). InGaAs and PbS devices are more suitable though less sensitive than CCDs. In certain diode array NIRS instruments, both silicon-based and InGaAs detectors are employed in the same instrument. Such instruments can record both UV-visible and NIR spectra 'simultaneously'.

6.3. Choice of wavelengths

The NIR-spectrum is between 700 and 2500 nm. Reflectance spectroscopy uses wavelengths between 1100 and 2500 nm, although the extremes of this range are not often used. This region of the infrared spectrum gives results which have a signal: noise ratio of about 10,000: 1 and are attenuated enough so that samples do not have to be diluted and possible non-linearity caused by strong absorbances is less likely.

Table 6.1. Wavelengths used in the application of NIR-spectroscopy

S.No.	Analysis	Wavelength range (nm)
1.	Protein content in forages	2100 - 2164
2.	Protein content in grass	1536 - 2236
3.	Fibre content in forages	1555 - 1674
4.	Cellulose content in grass	1320 - 2044
5.	ME content of fodder	1658 - 1668

Reflectance in the NIR- spectrum represents the chemical structure of the sample. In particular it indicates the presence of chemical bonds and functional groups (C-H, O-H, N-H).

Table 6.2. NIR-wavelengths and their association with chemical structures

S.No.	Wavelength range (nm)	Chemical entity
1.	1143	Lignin
2.	1660-1670, 1720-1730, 2100-2200	Condensed tannins
3.	1930	Water
4.	1960, 2180	Protein
5.	2140, 2180	Peptide bonds
6.	2088, 2410-2460	Cellulose
7.	2380	Hemicellulose
8.	2461	Starch

6.4. Technical errors in near infrared-spectroscopy

Although NIR-spectroscopy is rapid and technically simple to carry out, there are many sources of error. These contribute to error in both the calibration and validation processes. Among them, error regarding to variation in water content of sample and particle size are particularly important.

Table 6.3. Error in NIR-spectroscopy

S.No.	Error	Sample factor
1.	Instrument noise	Variations in water content
2.	Stray light	Bulk density, texture, packing characteristics
3.	Non-linearity of signal	Sample temperature
4.	Static electricity	Subsampling procedures
5.	Instrument temperature control	Mean particle size, particle size distribution
6.	Fluctuations in power supply	Mixing after preparation
7.	Instrument geometry cell window characteristics	Sample storage

6.5. Procedure (Pasquini, 2003)

i) Prepare samples by the same method as the calibration samples were prepared.

ii) For best results run instrument (but not lamp) continuously. If instrument is cold, warm-up time should be 1 hr.

iii) Clean sample holder with a camel hair brush or vacuum. Additional cleaning may be done with soft tissue or lint-free cloth. Glass should be free of finger prints and foreign material.

iv) Load NIR sample cup placing one scoop of forage (previously dried to 90-95% dry matter or greater, ground with cyclone mill to pass 1 mm screen, thoroughly mixed) on each third of the glass surface to ensure that portions of different subsamples are scanned.

v) Press back into holder so that sample is firmly pressed against window.

vi) If any abnormality appears in window, remove back and repeat process. Consistency in sample handling, preparation, and cell packing is crucial to success.

vii) Scan sample, collect spectra, and process data.

Prediction is made by direct comparison to calibration. No additional calculations. If calibrations were made using reference values on a DM basis, NIR-spectroscopy results will be expressed on a DM basis.

6.6. Precautions

i) NIR instrument should be maintained in a dust-free environment. Clean or change filter monthly. Clean ceramic standard and drawer assembly monthly.

ii) Never touch or clean grating.

iii) NIR instrument should be maintained in a stable-temperature (25 °C) room with controlled humidity (60%). Room should be free from vibration and have stable and dedicated electrical current.

iv) Sample must be dried and ground by the same methods as those samples used to develop the calibration equation.

v) Spectrophotometer reads only a fraction of 1 mm depth of material touching glass of sample container. Therefore container must be loaded carefully with different subsample in each quadrant to make spectral reading more representative of entire sample.

6.7. Advantages of near infrared-spectroscopy

i) Rapid, as minimal or no sample preparation necessary.

ii) High throughput makes NIR-spectroscopy a cheap technique on a sample basis.

iii) Very accurate and highly precised.

iv) Non-destructive technique, allows simultaneous measurement of several parameters.

v) Environmentally friendly: no reagents, no chemical waste.

6.8. Limitations of near infrared-spectroscopy

i) Suitable for major feed components, not for minor components.

ii) Great care needed in developing calibrations as these are matrix specific.

iii) Complexity in choice of data treatment is confusing for the novice.

iv) Calibration procedures are time consuming and only worthwhile for subsequent analysis of large sample numbers.

v) High instrument costs.

❐❐❐

7

Determination of Energy Content

7.1. Procedure for determination of gross energy of sample by bomb calorimeter 60

7.2. Limitations of bomb calorimeter 62

The gross energy (GE) is the amount of heat produced from unit feed when it is completely burnt down to its ultimate oxidation products (CO_2 and H_2O). The feed is burnt is a closed container and heat produced from it is measured by bomb calorimeter. The most common type of calorimeter is the oxygen bomb calorimeter. The calorific value as determined in an oxygen bomb calorimeter is measured by a substitution procedure in which the heat obtained from the sample is compared with the heat obtained from combustion of a similar amount of benzoic acid whose calorific value is known. The energy released by this combustion is absorbed within the calorimeter and the resulting temperature change within the absorbing medium is noted. The calorific value of the sample is calculated by multiplying the temperature rise in the calorimeter by a previously determined energy equivalent determined from previous tests with a standardizing material.

Bomb calorimetry is used to determine the enthalpy of combustion, $D_{comb}H$, for hydrocarbons. Since combustion reactions are usually exothermic (give off heat), $D_{comb}H$ is typically negative. The bomb calorimeter consists primarily of the sample, oxygen, the stainless steel bomb, and water. The dewar prevents heat flow from the calorimeter to the rest of the universe.

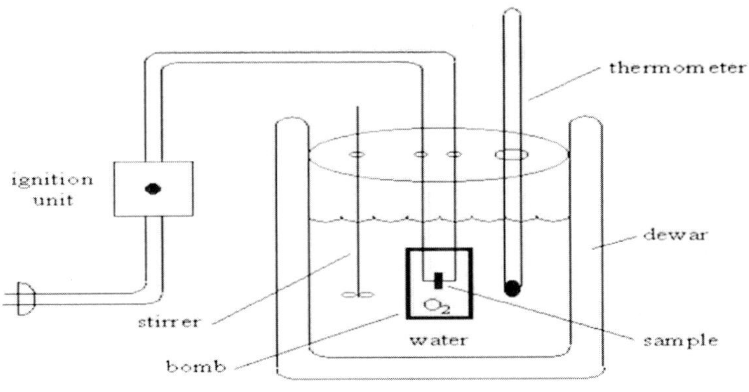

Figure 7.1. Diagram of bomb calorimeter

7.1. Procedure for determination of gross energy of sample by bomb calorimeter

There are following steps while estimating GE value of feedstuffs and faeces using bomb calorimeter (AOAC, 1995):

1. Filling the bomb calorimeter

i) Press the material (feed or excreta) into a tablet weighing 0.5-1.0 g.

ii) Weigh the material, wrap it in weighted cigarette paper and secure with 20 cm long thread of uniform thickness.

iii) Connect a 10 cm platinum wire of stainless steel wire to the two electrodes of the bomb.

iv) Place the tablet in the crucible and tie the thread to platinum wire to carry the flame to the tablet in the crucible.

v) Add about 10 ml of distilled water to the bomb.

vi) Put the assembly in the bomb, tighten the cap and fill oxygen into the bomb through its inlet value up to 25 lbs pressure per square inch.

2. Adjustment of water temperature in the pail

Add 2000 ml of distilled water to the pail and keep it in proper position in the outer jacket. Keep the temperature of the outer jacket 5-6 ^{o}F higher than the water taken in the pail.

3. Assembling the calorimeter

Place the bomb in the pail and connect with mains of the switch box. Place the stir, thermometer and lid of the calorimeter in their proper position.

4. Ignition

Switch on the stirrer and record the initial temperature after about five minutes. Ignite the bomb by pressing the push button for 3-4 seconds. Record the final temperature after it is constant for 2 to 3 minutes.

5. Dissembling the calorimeter

Remove the connecting wires, thermometer, stirrer and covering lids. Take out the bomb and release slowly the gas pressure inside the bomb. Open the bomb; wash all interior surfaces with a jet of distilled water. Collect the washings in 250 ml beaker for estimation of H_2SO_4 and HNO_3 formed form sulphur and nitrogen present in the test sample.

6. Measurement of heat of combination

Calculate heat of combustion from the rise in temperature and water equivalent (mentioned below). Correct it for the formation of acids.

7. Correction for the acid formation

i) Boil the washings collected in the beaker.

ii) Cool and titrate against N/10 barium hydroxide using phenolphthalein indicator.

iii) Add to it 20 ml N/10 sodium carbonate solution and boil.

iv) Cool the contents filter and give 3 washing wash with hot distilled water.

v) Titrate the washings against N/10 HCL using methyl orange indicator.

vi) Calculate the heat liberated by H_2SO_4 and HNO_3 using the following factors:

1ml N/10 $Ba(OH)_2$ = 3.60 cal

1 ml N/10 Na_2CO_3 = 1.43 cal

8. Determination of water equivalent

Use benzoic acid (dried over P_2O_5) which is a standard material having heat of combustion 6319 cal/g. Compute water equivalent of the calorimeter from the following equation:

$$W = \frac{H \times M + C1 + C2 + C3}{T}$$

Where, W is the water equivalent of calorimeter (cal/°F), H is the heat of combustion of standard benzoic acid (cal/g; 6319), M is the weight of benzoic acid (g), T is the rise in temperature of water of the pail, C1 and C2 are the correction for heat combustion (cal) of H_2SO_4 and HNO_3, respectively and C3 is the heat of combustion of used wire, paper and thread (heat of combustion of paper, thread and fuse wire may be taken as 3234 cal/g, 3962 cal/g and 1400 cal/g, respectively).

9. Calculation

$$\text{Gross heat of combustion (cal/g)} = \frac{T \times W + (C1 + C2 + C3)}{M}$$

Where, T is the rise in temperature, W is the water equivalent, M is the weight of substance, C1 and C2 are the correction for heat combustion (cal) of H_2SO4 and HNO_3, respectively and C3 is the heat of combustion of used wire, paper and thread.

7.2. Limitations of bomb calorimeter

i) Although bomb calorimeters in laboratories are insulated to minimize these loses, heat loss cannot, of course, be eradicated entirely.

ii) Moreover, the reactants in the calorimeter may not be well-mixed, which leads to uneven heating and another possible source of error in your measurements.

iii) Very slowly reaction like oxidation of iron to form rust would be very difficult to study with a calorimeter.

❑❑❑

8

Fatty Acid Analysis

8.1. Fatty acid analysis of feed by gas liquid chromatography-method 63

8.2. Milk fatty acid analysis by gas chromatography-method 65

The diet of farm animals has been traditionally low in fat, especially in herbivores; not more than 2 to 5 % of digestible energy. It has been known for some time that fat supplements can enhance productive performance in cattle, pigs and poultry, and there is currently much interest in optimizing the amount and type of fat in the diets of farm animals. The fatty acid profile of the feedstuff influences the fatty acid profile of the tissues. The EE fraction of plants, because it contains numerous nonnutritive substances, is not a nutritionally uniform fraction, whereas fatty acids constitute a uniform fraction that can be measured. The fatty acid composition in feedstuffs and milk should be analyzed more accurately by gas liquid chromatography (GLC) and gas chromatography (GC), respectively.

8.1. Fatty acid analysis of feed by gas liquid chromatography -method

Procedure

Steps in fatty acid analysis by chromatographic methods include Saponification, acidification, methylation, analysis and calculation (Sukhija and Palmquist, 1988).

1. Saponification

Take 50 to 500 mg of finely grind freeze dried sample of faeces or forage or feed to a 100 ml conical flask, add 5 ml of ethanol and 5 N sodium hydroxide solutions. Shake well and cover with foil. Place in oven at 80 °C for 1.5 to 2 hrs and then allow cooling.

2. Acidification

Add 3 ml of 5 N hydrochloric acid and invert test tube with care. pH must be checked for each sample using pH paper till acid (must be pink). When sample has cooled sufficiently. Extract fatty acids with 4 ml of petroleum ether, shake well, and pipette the supernatant into a labelled 15 ml test tube. Repeat above step - pooling the extracts. Evaporate pooled extracts to dryness in a warm water bath under a stream of nitrogen.

3. Methylation

To the dried sample add 3 ml of 1% sulphuric acid in methanol. Reflux on a heating block at 50 to 60 °C for 1.5 hrs. Add 3 ml of 5% NaCl (salt solution). Add 3 ml of petroleum ether (boiling range 40 to 60 °C). Cool, shake well and centrifuge and decant supernatant into GLC vial.

4. Operating conditions of GLC

1.	Injector temperature	20-50 °C higher than the column
2.	Oven temperature	220 °C
3.	Column	12-15 % ethylene glycol succinate on 100/ 120 mesh gas chrom P (2m x 4 mm, at 180 °C)
4.	Detector	Flame ionization detector (FID)
5.	Carrier gas	Inert gas (nitrogen, helium, argon)
6.	Auxillary gas	Hydrogen (99% purity)
7.	Reference standards	A mixture of methyl esters of known purity preferably similar to the fatty matter being analyzed

5. GLC analysis

Determine retention times and quantitative correction factors to be applied for the range of fatty acids to be run. Determine recovery of a fatty acid standard (e.g., 16:0 or 18:0) by weighing 20 to 50 mg of pure standard; add internal standard and run as for unknowns. Recoveries for duplicate analyses should be 100 ± 5% for both samples.

Total FA (mg/g) = sum of areas for all FA peaks compared to area for standard

Where, FA is the fatty acid. Report as mg of fatty acid/g of dry sample.

8.2. Milk fatty acid analysis by gas chromatography-method

Procedure

1. Saponification

   Pipette out 2 ml of a thoroughly mix milk sample into a 25 ml stoppered test tube, add 1 ml of ethanol and 5 N NaOH. Shake well and cover with foil. Place in oven at 80 °C for 1.5 to 2 hrs. Remove from oven and allow to cool.

2. Acidification

   For acidification, add 2 ml of 5 N HCl in above content in a test tube. Invert test tube with care and follow procedure as in 8.1.

3. Methylation (see 8.1)

4. Operating conditions of GC

1.	Oven profile	50 °C for 1 minute, then 25 °C/minute to 200 °C, then 3 °C/minute to 230 °C for 23 minutes
2.	Run time	40 minutes
3.	Detector	Flame ionization detector (FID)
4.	Injector temperature	250 °C
5.	Carrier gas	Helium
6.	Equilibrium time	0.5 minutes

5. GC analysis

   The sample fatty acid concentrations were calculated according to Joseph and Ackman (1992), using the equation:

$$C(mg/g) = \frac{Ax \times Ms \times Trf}{A \times Ma \times Fct}$$

Where, C is the concentration of fatty acid in sample, Ax is the area of fatty acid methyl esters (FAMEs), Ms is the internal standard mass added to the sample (mg), Trf is the theoretical response factor of FAMEs and Fct is the conversion factor to express the results in mg fatty acids/g total lipid.

□□□

9

Amino Acid Analysis

9.1. Amino acid analysis by non oxidized hydrolysis-method 67

9.2. Amino acid analysis by oxidized hydrolysis-method 68

Amino acids are building block of protein and may be grouped according to their transport affinities or essential role in animal nutrition or on the basis of catabolic fate of the carbon skeleton. Additional subsets are also recognized, based on common structural features. Leucine, isoleucine and valine are referred to as the branched chain amino acids (BCAA), whereas phenylalanine and tyrosine are categorized as the aromatic amino acids. Assessments of requirements for sulphur amino acids (SAA) are invariably based on a summation of methionine, cysteine and cystine needs, but it will be recalled that homocysteine is another member of this group. Another subset, the excitatory amino acids, includes glutamate and aspartate.

9.1. Amino acid analysis by non oxidized hydrolysis-method

Non oxidized method is used for the quantitative determination of amino acids in materials such as grain, feedstuff, milk, etc., which do not just consist of pure protein.

Procedure (Garg *et el.*, 2013)

i) Accurately weigh 200 mg of sample into a 250 ml round bottom flask. Add 2 glass beads.

ii) Add 160 ml HCl (6N) heat at 110°c for 23 hrs.

iii) Filter solution into a 250 ml measuring cylinder and make it upto 200 ml with de-ionised water.

iv) Take a 50 ml aliquot, place it into a 250 ml round bottom flask, and remove the acid using a rotary evaporator connected to a vacuum pump (water bath temperature 60 °C).

v) Rinse the residue twice with de-ionized water and evaporate to dryness.

vi) Store 50 ml in a specimen jar in case you need to repeat the procedure discard once you are happy with the results.

vii) Pipette 5 ml of diluting buffer into the residue, and transfer to a plastic scintillation vial.

viii) Filter about 0.5 ml through a 2 um filter, into a vial, so that it is ready to be used, with the appropriate buffer dilution. The samples are run under the "Hydrolysis program".

ix) The dilution is worked out according to the nitrogen % of the sample (the higher the nitrogen content the higher the dilution).

9.2. Amino acid analysis by oxidized hydrolysis-method

This method is used for the quantitative determination of cystine and methionine, (both acids must be converted into their stable oxidized forms using performic acid) to convert them to cysteic acid and methionine sulphone. During the oxidation tyrosine and histidine will be almost completely destroyed.

Reagents

i) Performic acid/hydrogen peroxide oxidation mixture:

To make	10 ml	20 ml	30 ml
Hydrogen peroxide 30%	1 ml	2 ml	3 ml
Performic acid 88%	9 ml	18 ml	27 ml
Liquid phenol	50 mg	100 mg	150 mg

Weigh the liquid phenol into a 50 or 100 ml conical flask, then add the other two reagents and mix, incubate for 1 hr at 30 °C, using a water bath.

ii) Sodium disulphite.

iii) 6 N Hydrochloric acid + phenol: (50 ml 6 N HCl, containing 50 mg phenol).

iv) Lithium citrate buffer: pH 2.20.

Procedure (Garg *et al.*, 2013)

i) Weigh 100 mg of sample into a 100 ml round bottom flask, and place them with enough ice to cover a third of the flask.

ii) Prepare the oxidation mixture and cool it together with the samples in ice.

iii) Add 5 ml of solution to each sample and swirl the flask to mix in the solution.

iv) Cover each flask with parafilm, and leave in the fridge for 16 hrs. This is where the oxidation occurs.

v) To stop the reaction, add 840 mg of sodium bisulphate.

vi) The hydrolysis is performed with 60 ml of 6 N HCl containing 60 mg phenol, add boiling chips, and reflux at 110 °C for 23 hrs.

vii) Filter solution into a 100 ml measuring cylinder, make it up to 100 ml with de-ionised water.

viii) Take a 50 ml aliquot, place it into a 250 ml round bottom flask, and remove the acid using a rotary evaporator connected to a vacuum pump (water bath temperature 60 °C). Rinse the residue twice with de-ionised water and evaporate.

ix) Store 50 ml into a specimen jar in case you need to repeat the procedure, discard once you are happy with the results.

x) Pipette 5 ml of diluting buffer into the residue, and transfer to a plastic scintillation vial.

xi) Filter about 0.5 ml through a 2 μm filter, into a vial, so that it is ready to be used, with the appropriate buffer dilution.

xii) The samples are run under the "Hydrolysis program".

□□□

10

Vitamin Analysis

10.1. Determination of vitamin A by high performance liquid chromatography-method 71
10.2. Determination of vitamin E by high performance liquid chromatography-method 75
10.3. Determination of vitamin D_3 by high performance liquid chromatography-method 76

Vitamins, a group of complex organic compounds that are present in minute amounts in natural foodstuffs, are essential for normal metabolism, and a lack of these compounds in the diet causes deficiency diseases. To date, 15 vitamins have been identified and classified as either fat (vitamin A, D, E and K) or water-soluble (vitamin B-complex and C). Separate methods based on reversed-phase high performance liquid chromatography (HPLC) for the determination of vitamins were proposed.

10.1. Determination of vitamin A by high performance liquid chromatography-method

The sample is saponified with ethanolic potassium hydroxide solution and the vitamin A is extracted into light petroleum. The light petroleum is removed by evaporation and the residue is dissolved in 2-propanol. The vitamin A concentration in the 2-propanol extract is determined by reverse-phase liquid chromatography using conditions that give a single peak for all retinol isomers.

Procedure (IS 15120: 2002)

1. Saponification

   i) Weigh about 0.1 g sample in 1 l conical flask.

ii) Add 200 ml of ethanol. Swirl the flask.

iii) Add 2 ml of sodium ascorbate and 50 ml of potassium hydroxide solution and mix by swirling.

iv) Fit a reflux condenser to the flask and immerse the flask in the boiling water bath.

v) Allow the contents of the flask to reflux for 60 minutes.

vi) Remove and cool the flask to room temperature as rapidly as possible under a stream of cold water.

2. Extraction of vitamin A

i) Transfer the contents of the flask to extraction cylinder.

ii) Rinse the flask with two 25 ml portions of ethanol and transfer the rinsing to cylinder.

iii) Repeat the rinsing of the flask with two 125 ml of petroleum and one 250 ml of water, each time transferring the rinsing to the cylinder.

iv) Stopper the cylinder and shake well for 1 minute.

v) Cool under a stream of cold water while waiting for the two liquid phases to separate, before removing the stopper.

vi) When the layers have separated, remove the stopper, wash the sides of the stopper with a few ml of light petroleum and insert the adjustable tube, positioning the lower open end so that it is just above the level of the interface. By application of a slight pressure of inert gas to the side-arm tube, transfer the upper, light petroleum layer to a 1 l separating funnel.

vii) Add 125 ml petroleum to cylinder and shake for 1 minute.

viii) Allow the layers to separate and transfer the upper layer to the separating funnel using the adjustable tube. Repeat above step again.

ix) Wash the combined light petroleum extracts with four 100 ml portions of water using at first only gentle inversion then only gentle shaking in order to keep emulsion formation to a minimum.

x) Transfer the washed extract through a medium/fast filter paper containing 60 g of anhydrous sodium sulfate, into a flask suitable for vacuum evaporation.

xi) Rinse the separating funnel with two 20 ml of light petroleum and add rinsing, through the filter to the evaporation flask.

xii) Wash the filter further with two 25 ml of light petroleum and collect the washings in the evaporation flask.

xiii) Evaporate the petroleum extract to dryness under vacuum at a temperature not exceeding 40 °C.

xiv) Restore atmospheric pressure by admitting inert gas.

3. HPLC analysis

i) Dissolve the residue in the minimum volume of 2-propanol and transfer quantitatively to a 20 ml volumetric flask.

ii) Rinse the evaporation flask with three small portions of 2-propanol, transferring the rinsing to the volumetric flask.

iii) Dilute to volume with 2-propanol and mix and inject 10 μl of the sample extract into HPLC.

iv) Calculate the peak area (1 IU of vitamin A is equal to 0.300 μg of all-trans-retinol. 1 IU of vitamin A is equal to 0.344 μg of all-trans-retinyl acetate).

4. Hydrolysis of all-trans-retinyl acetate for calibration

i) Prepare a solution of all-trans-retinyl acetate in ethanol, so that 1 ml contains approximately 15000 IU of vitamin A.

ii) Transfer 2.5 ml of this solution to a 150 ml flask.

iii) Add 20 ml of ethanol, 1 ml of potassium hydroxide and 5 ml of sodium solution.

iv) Fit a condenser to the flask. Immerse the flask in the boiling water bath and allow refluxing for 60 minutes. Cool the flask to room temperature under a stream of cold water and transfer the contents to a separating funnel.

v) Rinse the flask with 50 ml of water, followed by 25 ml of ethanol, adding the rinsing to the separating funnel. Extract the aqueous phase with 80 ml of petroleum followed with 50 ml portions of light petroleum.

vi) Combine petroleum extracts, and then wash with 50 ml portions of distilled water. Add 2 g of anhydrous sodium sulphate.

vii) Transfer petroleum extract to 250 ml volumetric flask and dilute to volume. The retinol concentration of this solution is approximately 150 IU/ml.

5. Standardization of retinol solution for calibration

i) Pipette 5 ml of above solution into a 50 ml volumetric flask and remove the solvent, at ambient temperature, with a stream of inert gas.

ii) Dissolve the residue in 2-propanol, and then dilute to volume with 2-propanol.

iii) Measure the absorbance of the solution, using 2-propanol as reference, at wavelengths of 310 nm, 325 nm and 334 nm. The absorbance values will be approximately 0.7 to 0.8. If necessary, an intermediate dilution may be used.

Using the following equation, calculate the corrected absorbance at 325 nm:

$$A_{325}, \text{corr} = 6.815 \times A_{325} - 2.555 \times A_{310} - 4.26 \times A_{334}$$

If $A_{325,corr} / A_{325}$ is less than 0.97, use the value of A_{325},corr for the standardization; otherwise use $A_{325.}$ The retinol concentration of solution 1 is given by:

$$\text{Concentration (IU/ml)} = A_{325} \times 183 \text{ IU/ml, or}$$

$$\text{Concentration (IU/ml)} = A_{325}, \text{corr} \times 183 \text{ IU/ml}$$

6. Preparation of a retinol standard for chromatography

i) Prepare a retinol solution in 2-propanol (for each 1000 IU of vitamin A/kg of sample, a retinol concentration of 2.5 IU/ml is expected in the extract).

ii) Evaporate an aliquot volume of solution to dryness at ambient temperature with a stream of inert gas. Dissolve the residue in the appropriate volume of 2-propanol to provide the required retinol concentration and mix it. If necessary, filter the standard solution through a membrane filter.

iii) For calibration purposes, a standard solution of vitamin A (retinol) in 2-propanol prepared by diluting a stock standard solution of all-trans-retinol made by dissolving an appropriate quantity of all-trans-retinol standard substance directly in 2-propanol may be used.

iv) Check the vitamin A standard by measuring the absorbance of the standard solution in quartz cells at wavelengths of 300 nm, 325 nm, 350 nm and 370 nm against 2-propanol as reference. Determine the A/A_{325} ratio at each of the wavelengths for all-trans-retinol. If the ratio does not exceed 0.602, 0.432 and 0.093 at 300 nm, 350 nm and 370 nm, respectively, the standard substance is suitable for use.

Calculation

Calculate the numerical value of the vitamin A content of the test sample by the equation.

$$wA = 200{,}000 \times \frac{c}{m}$$

Where, wA is the numerical value of the vitamin A content of the test sample, in IU/kg, c is the numerical value of the retinol concentration of the extract, in IU/ml and m is the numerical value of the mass of the test sample, in g.

10.2. Determination of vitamin E by high performance liquid chromatography-method

Procedure (Chawla and Kaur, 2001)

1.Extraction

i) Saponify about 1 g feed sample with 10 ml of 95% ethanol and 2 ml of 60% KOH in 50 ml conical flask.

ii) Keep the content on the boiling water both till one or two bubbles appears.

iii) Cool it by ice bath for 5 minutes and add 10 ml of petroleum ether.

iv) Shake the contents for 15 minutes in water bath at 39 °C and collect the extract in the vial. Repeat the same for three times.

v) Collect pooled ether extract and treat with 10 ml of 0.5 N KOH in a separating funnel.

vi) Wash the solution with distilled water for three times to remove the excess alkali.

vii) Finally collect ether and filter through sodium sulfate. Dry the EE under nitrogen gas.

viii) Residue is ready for injection to HPLC.

2. Operating conditions of HPLC

1.	Mobile phase	Acetonitrile: tetrahydrofuran: water (47:42:11)
2.	Flow rate	1.5 ml/minute
3.	Column	C 18 ODS (150 × 40 mm)
4.	Oven temperature	17 °C
5.	Detector	UV/PDA
6.	Wave length for vitamin E	290 nm
7.	Total run time	6 minutes

Calculations

$$\text{Vitamin E}(\mu g/g) = \frac{Ve \times SA \times SDC}{Vi \times SdA} \times \text{Purity of vitamin}$$

Where, Ve is the volume in which dried was dissolved, SA is the sample area from peak, SdC is the standard concentration of vitamin E, Vi is the volume injected and SdA is the standard area from the peak.

10.3. Determination of vitamin D_3 by high performance liquid chromatography-method

Procedure (Eirenmiller and Landen, 1998)

1. Extraction

i) Add about 1 g feed sample with 5 ml diethyl ether and keep it in freezer with acetone containing beaker till the lower portion freezes.

ii) Collect the supernatant in another vial. Repeat the same for three times.

iii) Add 4 ml mixture of dichloromethane and methanol (3:1) in the collected supernatant of each vial.

iv) Collect again supernatant from above mixture and treat with 0.1 M of phosphate buffer.

v) The supernatant of EE is collected and dried under nitrogen gas.

vi) Residue is ready for HPLC injection.

2. Operating conditions of HPLC

1.	Mobile phase	Acetonitrile (100%)
2.	Flow rate	2 ml/minute
3.	Column	C 18 ODS (150 × 40 mm)
4.	Oven temperature	25 °C
5.	Detector	UV/PDA
6.	Wave length	265 nm
7.	Total run time	10 minutes

Calculations

$$\text{Vitamin D3} (\mu g/g) = \frac{Ve \times SA \times SDC}{Vi \times SdA} \times \text{Purity of vitamin}$$

Where, Ve is the volume in which dried was dissolved, SA is the sample area from peak, SdC is the standard concentration of vitamin D3, Vi is the volume injected and SdA is the standard area from the peak.

❑❑❑

11

Biological Methods for Feed and Fodder Evaluation

Nutritive value of feeds is determined by a number of factors. These factors are generally measurable in the case of the animal as digestibility and intake. Digestibility is simply a measure of the availability of food nutrients. When digestibility is combined with intake data, one can make a rather accurate prediction of overall nutritive value and, hence, the potential production a given feed can support. There are following three biological methods used for evaluation of feeds and fodders.

1. Feed and fodder evaluation by *in vivo* method
2. Feed and fodder evaluation by *in sacco* method
3. Feed and fodder evaluation by *in vitro* method

11.1. Feed and fodder evaluation by *in vivo* method

Feed and fodder evaluated more precisely by conducting digestion and metabolism trial (*in vivo* method). The conventional digestion trial is the most reliable method of measuring the digestibility of a feedstuff. Unfortunately, however, it is somewhat time consuming, tedious, and costly. Basically, the feed in question is fed in known quantities to an animal. The animal is restrained in an individual cage so that a quantitative collection of faeces can be made. Accurate records of feed intake, refusals and fecal output are kept, and a subsample of each is retained for analysis. When estimates of nitrogen balance are desired, urine output also is measured. Digestion trial is carried out to evaluate the utilization of feedstuffs or nutrients. A metabolism trial is conducted to calculate balance of nutrients retained in the body. Samples of feed offered, residue left and faeces voided are collected during digestion trial while urine (milk in lactating animals) along with feed offered, residue left and faeces voided are collected during metabolism trial.

1. Principle

Weighed amount of experimental feed is fed to animal for a definite period of time and the excreta resulting there from are collected quantitatively for chemical analysis. By knowing the proximate principles in feed and faeces, digestion coefficients of nutrients can be calculated. If we analyze the urine and products such as milk or wool the amount of source of nutrients absorbed and retained in the body or stored as a product may be calculated by difference.

2. Grouping of animals

The animals selected for experiment should be of the same breed, sex, age and body weight. Animals should be healthy and free from parasites. Male animals are preferred to females because it is easier to collect faeces and urine separately.

3. Feeding and watering

i) Experimental animal should be fed at the same time each day early in the morning at about 9 A.M. The amount of experimental ration should be exactly weighed.

ii) Experimental animal should be allowed to drink clean and wholesome water at least 3 times a day in winter season and 4 to 6 times in summer season.

iii) If trace mineral or Ca and P balance studies are to be conducted then these contents should be analyzed in water.

4. Preliminary period

The test feed has to be fed daily in constant amounts, as per the requirements of the animal, for an extended period. This is called preliminary period. The purpose preliminary period is to make the gastrointestinal tract free of any indigestible material from the feed consumed prior to the start of the digestion trial. In monogastric animals such as pigs, digestion and evacuation are usually complete in 24 hrs after the test feed is ingested. In ruminants eating a roughage ration, the last residues may not be voided until 6 to 8 days have elapsed. So preliminary period of 2 to 3 days in monogastric and 7 to 14 days in ruminants is followed.

5. Collection period and sampling

Animals are transferred to cages or stalls and a 2 to 3 day adaptation period is allowed for their acclimatisation. This follows collection period of 7 to 10 days duration (5 to 7 day collection period is mostly followed). In general, the longer the period of collection the more accurate the results are, provided the stated amount of feed continues to be consumed regularly and completely, since the effect of periodic fluctuations is minimised. Quantitative collection of faeces and urine are done. Representative samples of feed offered, feed leftovers and faeces and urine voided are preserved and analysed for nutrient composition.

i) In the case of male animals, use of urine bags are advised, while faeces is collected manually and kept in the plastic buckets.

ii) In the case of female animals, polyethylene tube fitted in the urethral orifice and supported by adhesive tape fixed on the labia major is used for collection of urine.

iii) Daily (24 hrs) amount of faeces voided is recorded and $1/50^{th}$ total weight is taken for dry matter estimation and preserved daily in polythene bags.

iv) Another aliquot of faeces $1/100^{th}$ is carefully weighed in a water glass and transferred to a glass mortar and mixed with 5 ml 30% H_2SO_4 for mixing the nitrogen, the mixed sample is taken in wide mouth glass bottle.

v) Amount of faeces collected in the bottle during a period of 5 to 7 days is weighed and weight of H_2SO_4 added is deducted from the total weight so as to know the actual weight of faeces in the bottle.

vi) An aliquot $1/100^{th}$ is taken in the Kjeldahl flask for nitrogen estimation.

vii) If trace element in the urine is to be determined then another aliquot $1/100^{th}$ is taken in the glass bottles rinsed with glass distilled water and 1 ml of distilled 30% H_2SO_4 is added to each bottle so as to prevent fermentation.

6. Analysis

The representative samples of feed and fodder offered, residues left and faeces and urine voided during digestion/metabolism trial are analyzed for proximate composition (see 3), fibre fraction (see 4), energy value (see 7), mineral content (see 5), etc.

Calculation

$$DC(\%) = \frac{\text{Amount of the nutrient in feed consumed - Amount of the nutrient in faeces}}{\text{Amount of the nutrient in feed consumed}} \times 100$$

$$\text{Apparant digestibility}(\%) = \frac{\text{Amount consumed - Faecal excretion}}{\text{Amount consumed}} \times 100$$

$$\text{True digestibility}(\%) = \frac{\text{Amount consumed - (Faecal excretion - Metabolic losses)}}{\text{Amount consumed}} \times 100$$

Where, DC is the digestibility coefficient of a nutrient.

11.2. Feed and fodder evaluation by *in sacco* method

In sacco or semi- *in vivo* or nylon bag or *in situ* technique is another method of evaluation of feeds and fodders. The incubation of feeds in nylon bags inside the rumen is used to measure the degradation of the feedstuff. Degradability is expressed as loss of weight during incubation.

1. Procedure

i) Weigh 3 g of dried and ground feed (3 mm mesh size; 40-60 μm porosity; 14 × 9 cm diameter) in each nylon bag (Ms).

ii) Attach 3 to 5 bags to each plastic tube and insert in rumen. Up to 12 bags can be inserted in rumen for incubation time of 4, 8, 16, 24, 36, 48, 72 and 96 hrs (use at least three animals).

iii) Insert bags at different time intervals to take them out at the same time.

iv) Take out bags at different time intervals and put immediately in cold water to stop fermentation.

v) Washed bag under tap water (until wash water is clear).

vi) Dry bags in hot air oven at 50 °C for 24 hrs, followed by 1 hrs at 100 °C.

vii) Weigh residues (Mr).

viii) Proceed with NDF determination for residues as under 4.1.

Calculation

i) Calculation of DM degradability

$$\text{DM deg} = \frac{\text{DMs - DMr}}{\text{DMs}} \times 100$$

Where, DM deg is the DM degraded, DMs is the DM content of sample and DMr is the DM content of residue left.

ii) Calculation of digestibility

$$\text{Digestibility} = \frac{\text{NDFr}}{\text{DMr}} \times 100$$

Where, NDFr is the NDF of residues and DMr is the DM content of residue left.

2. Advantages of the techniques

i) Technique provide useful tool for initial evaluation of feeds and fodders, and is useful in screening, rapidly, large number of samples developed in forage breeding experiments.

ii) This technique is helpful to understand the rumen processes. It is possible to vary the factors within the bag or within the rumen.

iii) The effective rumen degradability of nutrient can be calculated.

3. Limitations of the techniques

i) The test feed in the nylon bag is not subjected to the total ruminal experience like mastication, rumination and passage.

ii) What is actually measured is the breakdown of material to a size small enough to leave the bag and not necessarily a complete degradation to simple chemical compounds.

11.3. Feed and fodder evaluation by *in vitro* method

In vitro digestibility techniques provide a quick, inexpensive, and precise prediction of *in vivo* or conventionally determined digestibility in ruminants. Essentially, the method simulates the processes that occur in the rumen. The preliminary screening of feed samples may be done by *in vitro* gas production technique give by Menke et al. (1979) and Menke and Steingass (1988). The fermentation will be conducted in glass syringes containing the substrate and buffered rumen fluid at various times of incubation. The rate and extent of gas production can be estimated by fitting modified Mitscherlich equation of Orskov and McDonald (1979) model of single exponential equation with and without lag phase to study the gas production kinetics of substrate.

1. Preparation of buffer media

All the solutions are prepared as per Menke and Steingass (1988). The composition of different solutions is given below.

a) Micro mineral solution

S.No.	Chemical	Amount
1.	Calcium chloride ($CaCl_2 . 2H_2O$)	13.2 g
2.	$MnCl_2 . 4H_2O$	10.0 g
3.	$CoCl_2 . 6H_2O$	1.0 g
4.	$FeCl_3 . 6H_2O$	8.0 g
	Dissolved in 100 ml of water	

b) Buffer solution

S.No.	Chemical	Amount
1.	NH_4HCO_3	4.0 g
2.	$NaHCO_3$	35.0 g
	Dissolved in 1000 ml of water	

c) Macro mineral solution

S.No.	Chemical	Amount
1.	Na_2HPO_4 anhydrous	5.7 g
2.	KH_2PO_4 anhydrous	6.2 g
3.	$MgSO_{4.} 7H_2O$	0.6 g

Dissolved in 1000 ml of water

d) Reduction solution

S.No.	Chemical	Amount
1.	1 N NaOH	2.0 ml
2.	$Na_2S. 9H_2O$	285.0 mg

Dissolved in 47.5 ml of water

e) Resazurine solution

All the solution may be prepared before the start of incubation except the reduction solution, which should be prepared freshly each time before the rumen fluid was collected. The solution will pour into a Woulff flask, mixed with a magnetic stirrer and warmed to 39 °C in a PVC water bath with digital thermostat in the following order:

S.No.	Solutions	Quantity (ml)
1.	Distilled water	365
2.	Micro mineral solution	0.1
3.	Buffer solution	183
4.	Macro mineral solution	183
5.	Reduction solution	38.8
6.	Rumen liquor	330
	Total volume	1099.9

CO_2 gas should be passed through the submerged tube in the Woulff flask continuously during buffer media preparation. On the day of incubation, the mixture of rumen liquor and particulate matter should be collected from the fistulated donor animal (before feeding) into pre warmed CO_2 filled thermos and carried to the laboratory. The rumen fluid must be bubbled with CO_2 gas for few minutes and then add it to the buffer media when it will become colorless. All handling of rumen liquor should be done under continuous flushing with CO_2.

2. Filling of syringes and incubation

Dispense 30 ml buffered fluid to each syringe by an automatic dispenser. After recording initial volume, place the syringes in the incubator maintained at 39 °C. The gas production may be recorded at 0, 3, 6, 9, 12, 18, 24, 36, 48, 72 and 96 hrs of incubation and syringes should be shaken by hand intermittently. If the gas volume exceed 80 ml mark gas should be released. The fermentation will be terminated after 96 hrs of incubation. The fermentation kinetics can be estimated by means of nonlinear regression as follows:

$$Y = b \times (1\text{-}e^{-ct})$$

$$Y = b \times (1\text{-}e^{-c \times (t-L)})$$

Where, Y is the gas production (ml) at time t, b is the potential gas production (ml), c is the fractional rate of fermentation and L is the discrete lag time (h).

The average fermentation rate (ml gas/h) was defined as the average gas production rate between the start of incubation and the time at which the cumulative gas production was half of its asymptotic value, and may be calculates as:

$$\text{Rate} = b\ [c/2\ (\ln 2 + cxl)]$$

Substrate specific times were defined by the half time (T1/2) of asymptotic gas production and calculated as:

$$T1/2 = \ln 2/c$$

Voluntary feed intake potential (g DM/ kg $BW^{0.75}$) can be calculated from *in vitro* gas production kinetics parameters using the equation of Makkar et al. (1993) as follows:

$$\text{Intake (g DM/kg } BW^{0.75}) = 18.90 + 0.23\ (a+b) + 687 \times c + 0.11\ CP$$

3. Truly degradable DM and OM and efficiency of microbial biomass production

After the preliminary screening of the feed sample on the basis of gas production at half time (T1/2), true degradability of DM (TDDM) and OM (TDOM) and microbial biomass production (MBP) may be determined by incubating the substrate upto half time (T1/2) and/or 24 hrs. The content of syringes is to be transferred to 500 ml spoutless beakers by repeated washing with neutral detergent solution without sodium sulphate. The content is refluxed for 1 h and the residue may be recovered in pretarred filter crucibles. After drying the crucibles (with residue) to constant weigh, ignited at 450 °C for 30 minutes. TDDM, TDOM, OMD and MBP may be calculated as follows:

TDDM = Feed (DM) incubated – residue (DM)

TDOM = Feed (OM) incubated – residue (OM)

OM% = 14.88 + 0.889 × net gas production (24 hrs) + 0.45 × CP (% DM)

MBP = TDOM – (2.2 × net gas volume)

4. Partitioning factor (F) and metabolizable energy (ME) calculation

PF may be calculated as the ratio of mg of TDOM to ml of gas thereby produced. ME may be estimated from the gas volume as suggested by Menke and Steingass (1988) using the equation:

ME (MJ/kg DM) = 2.20 + 0.136 × gas (ml 200/mg DM) + 0.0057 × CP (% DM)

11.4. RUSITEC Technique

The technique is called as RUSITEC (Rumen simulation technique) that can replace cattle used in experiments. RUSITEC consist of water bath, reaction vessel, perforated cage, effluent bottle, gas bag, saliva tank, peristaltic pump, water heater, control panel. It is basically an *in vitro* semi continuous culture system. It simulates heterogeneous rumen under simplified conditions. Accurately weighed 10 g of feed/fodder to be tested for their nutritive value is placed in the perforated cage along with the inoculum (microbes) from the donor animal (input) in the reaction vessel. The amount of solid material that leaves the vessels each day is known as it is taken out manually. The output or the end product of fermentation (VFA, CH_4 and CO_2) can be determined from the effluent. The complete unit has eight reaction vessels, each representing a cow. Thus it is sufficient enough to conduct a valid number of replication to derive meaningful conclusion in research work.

❑❑❑

12

Enteric Methane Measurement in Ruminants

12.1. Measuring enteric methane production by using respiration chamber 89

12.2. Measuring enteric methane production by sulphur hexafluoride tracer technique 90

12.3. *In vitro* gas production technique 94

12.4. Methane determination by carbon dioxide technique 96

Methane (CH_4) is the major green house gas (GHG) produced from enteric fermentation during the normal digestive process of ruminants. CH_4 has a greenhouse potential 23 times that of CO_2. Interest in measuring enteric CH_4 emissions has moved from a focus on nutritional inefficiency to one of contributing to GHG concentrations in the atmosphere and climate change. Measurement of CH_4 emissions due to enteric fermentation must be also taken under conditions as close as possible to typical as found in farming systems. Methodologies for measuring CH_4 emissions range from animal respiration chambers to estimation of model techniques.

12.1. Measuring enteric methane production by using respiration chamber

The principle of the respiratory chamber is to collect exhaled CH_4 emissions from all sources of enteric fermentation (mouth, nostrils, and rectum) from the animal and to measure the concentration. Chambers are divided into two types, the closed-circuit and the open-circuit, with the latter being the dominating one. An air pump removes all air from the space through a flow meter and gas sensors in the open-circuit system. Each chamber is fitted with internal ventilation fans for efficient mixing of expired gases and incoming air. Air inlet is located at the front and an air outlet at the back. Fresh air to chamber is directly drawn from outside or through an air conditioning system to control humidity and temperature. The chamber is equipped with sensors for measuring relative humidity, temperature and barometric pressure. These allow air flow data to be adjusted for dry, standard temperature and pressure conditions. Outlet gas from each chamber is continuously sampled for analysis. Air flow is ducted via flexible polyurethane hoses. Air circulation is provided throughout the chambers at continuous but adjustable flow rates (usually 100-250 l/minute). The difference between the outgoing and incoming amount of CH_4 expresses the CH_4 emission.

12.2. Measuring enteric methane production by sulphur hexafluoride tracer technique

The main purpose of the method was to investigate energy efficacy in free ranging cattle, because it had been queried that results obtained in respiration chambers could not be applied to free ranging animals. The basic idea behind the method is that CH_4 emission can be measured if the emission rate of a tracer gas from the rumen is known. For this purpose a non-toxic, physiologically inert, stable gas is needed. Furthermore, the gas should mix with rumen air in the same way as CH_4. Sulphur hexafluoride (SF_6) was chosen, because it fulfills the above criteria, cheap, has an extremely low detection limit and is simple to analyze.

A. Principle

The SF_6 measurement technique measures the rate at which cattle release CH_4 using a tracer technique. A permeation device that release SF_6 at a known rate is placed in rumen. The animal is fitted with a sampling system such that ambient air from around the mouth and nostrils can be collected over an extended period of time. The air sample is then analyzed for CH_4 and SF_6 and these concentrations along with the known release rate allow calculation of the CH_4 emission rate.

B. Components of the system

The components of the system include a permeation device placed inside the rumen a halter that fits snugly around the cow's head, a PVC yoke that fits over the neck, capillary tubing for air transfer, a gas dilution system, and gas chromatographs for CH_4 and SF_6 determination.

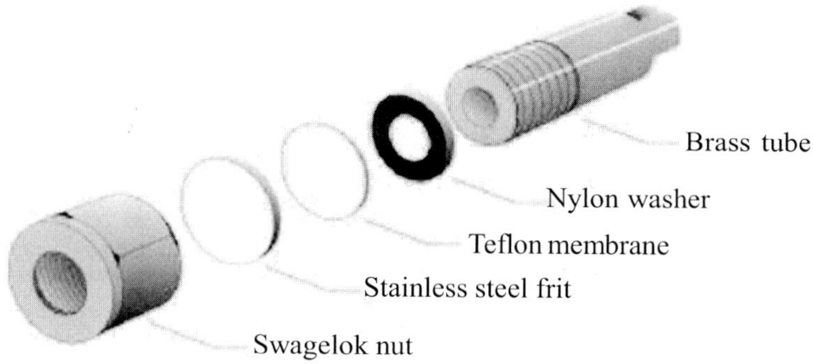

Figure 12.1. Components of permeation device

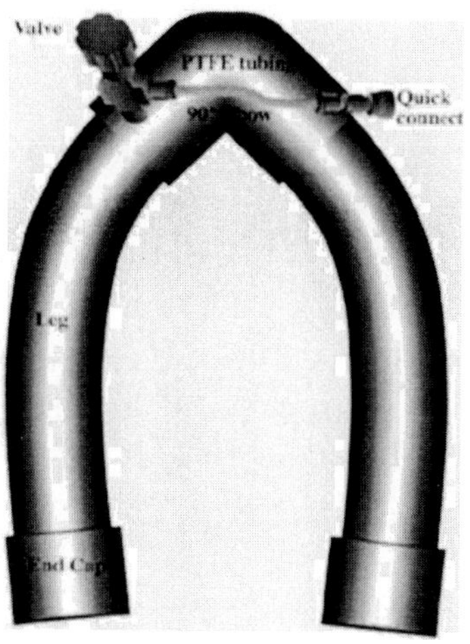

Figure 12.2. PVC collector canister (yoke) parts

C. Procedure

i) To charge the permeation tube with $SF_{6,}$ the nut, teflon window and frit are removed followed by immersion of the tube body in a cryogen such as liquid nitrogen. After the tube has reached the cryogen temperature, it is removed and any liquid is poured out of the cavity.

ii) Fill quickly the cavity of permeation tube with SF_6. The filling is accomplished by withdrawing about 60 cc of gaseous SF_6 in each of two plastic syringes. The needle is placed in the cavity of the permeation tube body and the plunger is slowly depressed by transfer the gaseous SF_6 into the permeation tube body cavity. The tube is quickly capped with teflon window, frit and nut following completion of the SF_6 transfer.

iii) Weigh permeation device. This procedure should provide a tube containing about 600 mg of SF_6.

iv) The tube should then be placed in a glass receptacle, in a 39 °C water bath. A small flow of clean N_2 gas is maintained to purge the glass receptacle of SF_6 emissions.

v) Weight of each tube should be taken weekly to determine the release rate of SF_6 (upto 5–6 weeks). Short sample integration periods (1 hr) may require only a short piece of tubing while longer periods (24 hrs) require much longer lengths of tubing.

vi) Assemble the PVC pieces, and allowing the glue to dry (12-24 hrs).

vii) Place the entire assembly into a 120-135 °C oven for 5-10 minutes. Keep checking the pipe by squeezing it until it is soft and pliable. Remove the pliable pipe and bend the legs into the desired position such that it should fit with cow's neck.

viii) Install the gas sampling valve and check the canister for leaks by pressurizing it with compressed air or nitrogen to 40 psi and then submerging it in water to watch for bubbles.

ix) Evacuate the canister by using vacuum pump.

x) After closing the valve on the canister, it is then ready to use.

xi) After the sample collection period has been completed, the canister is taken off the animal and connected to the dilution system and the final pressure recorded.

xii) Add N_2 slowly until the pressure in the canister is increased to about 1.2 atmospheric pressure. Another pressure reading is recorded to calculate the dilution factor.

xiii) Attached canister directly to the gas sampling valve in the GC via quick connects fittings and measure the CH_4 content.

D. Calculation

CH_4 concentration in the sampling canister is determined by GC. SF_6 is measured using a GC equipped with an electron capture detector (EID). The tracer method utilizes SF_6 to account for dilution as gases exiting the cow's mouth mix with ambient air. It is assumed that the SF_6 emission exactly simulates the CH_4 emission; thus, the dilution rates for SF_6 and CH_4 are identical. Mixing due to turbulent diffusion is much more important than molecular diffusion in the atmosphere. Similarly, gas transport from the rumen out of the mouth is dominated by forceful contractions and eructation so that molecular emission rate (QCH_4) can then be calculated from measured CH_4 and SF_6 concentrations and the known release rate of SF_6 (QSF_6):

$$(QCH4) = \frac{(QSF6) \times CH4}{(SF6)}$$

Background concentrations of CH_4 and SF_6 should be subtracted from the concentration of these species measured in the collection yoke. The background SF_6 concentrations are normally very small compared to yoke concentrations and therefore can usually be neglected.

E. Limitation of SF_6 technique

i) Very difficult to establish uniform release rate in permeation tube. Permeation tubes with high release rates give higher CH_4 emissions than tubes with low release rates. It is therefore recommended to use permeation tubes with nearly the same release rate when comparison of different treatments is needed.

ii) Measuring a representative background concentration under field condition can be difficult, because wind direction and other animals in the field can affect the concentrations.

iii) Inconsistency between CH_4 measurements determined in chambers and with SF_6 and within and between animal variations. Johnson *et al.* (2007) observed a 7% lower CH_4 emission with the SF_6 technique than with chambers with cattle, and this can partly be explained by the few percent of CH_4, which is lost via rectum.

12.3. *In vitro* gas production technique

The *in vitro* gas production technique (IVGPT) has been used to simulate ruminal fermentation of feedstuffs (Menke and Steingass, 1988). The basic principle of IVGPT is to ferment feed under controlled laboratory conditions employing natural rumen microbes. Feedstuffs subjected to different treatments, are incubated at 39 °C with a mixture of rumen fluid, buffer and minerals for a certain time period. The amount of total gas produced during incubation is measured and its composition analyzed, to obtain data on the *in vitro* production of CH_4. At the same time it is possible to determine *in vitro* degradation of the feedstuffs, making it possible to determine whether a reduction in CH_4 production is at the cost of total feed degradation. Various IVGPT systems have been employed for CH_4 determination as for example syringes, rusitec, closed vessel batch fermentations and lately fully automated systems. Depending on the system and other laboratory constraints it is possible to conduct up to several hundred parallel incubations at a time, which allows for sufficient amounts of repetitions in experiments to support statistically significant differences between treatments.

A. Solution

Table 12.1. Composition of different solutions

S.No.	Item	Amount
a) Macro-mineral solution		
1.	Na_2HPO_4	2.7 g
2.	KH_2PO_4	6.2 g
3.	$MgSO_4.7H_2O$	0.6 g
4.	Distilled water	1000 ml
b) Micro-mineral solution		
1.	$CaCl_2.2H_2O$	13.2 g
2.	$MnCl_2.4H_2O$	10.0 g
3.	$CoCl_2.6H_2O$	1.0 g
4.	$FeCl_2.6H_2O$	0.8 g
5.	Distilled water	100 ml
c) Buffer solution		
1.	NH_4HCO_3	4.0 g

2.	$NaHCO_3$	35.0 g
3.	Distilled water	1000 ml
d) Resazurine solution		
1.	Resazurine	100 mg
2.	Distilled water	100 ml
e) Reduction solution		
1.	NaOH (1N)	1.05 ml
2.	$Na_2S.9H_2O$	146.5 mg
3.	Distilled water	23.75 ml

Table 12.2. Composition of rumen inoculum

S.No.	Solution	Quantity
1.	Distilled water	365 ml
2.	Buffer	183 ml
3.	Macro-mineral solution	183 ml
4.	Micro-mineral solution	0.07 ml
5.	Resazurine	0.95 ml
6.	Reduction solution	1.6 ml
7.	Strained rumen liquor	330 ml
	Total	1063.62 ml

B. Procedure

i) Take 200 mg of substrate (samples) into 100 ml calibrated glass syringes with pistons lubricated with vaseline.

ii) Dispense 30 ml of buffered rumen fluid into each syringe containing the weighed diet samples.

iii) Close the clips on the silicon tube at the syringe tip.

iv) Gently shake the content of syringe. Open clips to remove gas by pushing the piston upwards to achieve complete gas removal.

v) Close the clips and record initial volume.

vi) Immediately place syringes in a thermostatically controlled shaking water bath at 39 °C.

vii) Three syringes containing 30 ml inoculum served as blanks.

viii) Complete incubation in triplicate within each run and the runs were replicated thrice.

Calculation

Record gas production at different hours of incubation. Evacuate gas samples in vials and go for to CH_4 analysis by using GC.

12.4. Methane determination by carbon dioxide technique

A newly developed method for estimating CH_4 emissions from livestock is based on the use of CO_2 as a tracer gas. Instead of using externally added SF_6, the naturally emitted CO_2 is used to quantify CH_4 emission. The CH_4 and CO_2 ratio in the production of air of the animal(s) is measured at regular intervals and combined with the calculated total daily CO_2 production of the animal(s). The measured feed intake can be converted to heat and there is a close relationship between heat and CO_2 production. Animals at maintenance are emits 1 l CO_2 per 21.5–22.0 KJ of heat produced. The relation between heat production and CO_2 production is partly related to the amount of fat deposited or mobilized and can in practice be as low as 20.0 KJ/l CO_2 when large amounts of feed carbohydrates are converted to fat as in high yielding dairy cows. The total CO_2 production from stables with different animals has likewise been determined by researchers working with ventilation.

The expired air from cattle contains CO_2 and CH_4 in concentrations 100 and 1000 times higher than the concentrations in atmospheric air, respectively. Therefore it is only necessary to have 5–10% of the animal's breath in the air being analyzed. This can easily be achieved in a stable. The method can potentially be developed for application to grazing cattle. As about 95% of CH_4 emissions from cows are excreted with expiration air, the small amounts excreted through the rectum can be ignored. The main disadvantage is that the CO_2 production of animals is influenced by the same things as the animals' requirement for energy. This means that the size, activity and production of the animal influences the amount of CO_2 produced. This is not of importance when for instance the quantitative effect of different feeds or supplements on the CH_4 production of different groups of equal animals is going to be established, but may produce larger errors when the quantitative CH_4 production is going to be established on an individual animal or on different groups of animals.

□□□

13

Rumen Liquor Analysis

13.1. Methods of rumen liquor collection 98
13.2. Examination of rumen fluid 100
13.3. Ruminal bacteria counting 103
13.4. Ruminal protozoa counting 104
13.5. Estimation of total volatile fatty acids 106
13.6. Determination of total nitrogen 107
13.7. Determination of trichloroacetic acid precipitable nitrogen 109
13.8. Determination of soluble nitrogen 110
13.9. Determination of ammonia nitrogen 110
13.10. Determination of lactic acid 110

Microbes in the rumino-reticulum includes bacteria, protozoa, fungi, archae and viruses. Bacteria, along with protozoa, are the predominant microbes and by mass account for 40-60% of total microbial matter in the rumen. They are categorized into several functional groups, such as fibrolytic, amylolytic, and proteolytic types, which preferentially digest structural carbohydrates, non-structural carbohydrates, and protein, respectively. Protozoa derive their nutrients through phagocytosis of other microbes, degrade and digest feed carbohydrates, especially starch sugars, and protein. Although protozoa are not essential for rumen functioning, their presence has pronounced effects. Ruminal fungi make up only 5-10% of microbes and are absent/lower on diets poor in fibre. Despite their low numbers, the fungi still occupy an important niche in the rumen because they hydrolyze some ester linkages between lignin and hemicellulose or cellulose, and help break down digesta particles. The analysis of ruminal fluid and its key examination are carried out, because it is an immense source of major beneficial organisms. The observation of rumen fluid is done to analyze the activity of the ruminant as well as the diagnosis of diseases of the fore stomach.

13.1. Methods of rumen liquor collection

Samples should be collected at a time when rumen pH is likely to be near the lowest point of the day. If the ration is fed as separate components, rumen liquor collection should be performed between 2 to 4 hrs after the cow is offered the primary concentrate meal of the day. If the ration is fed as a total mixed ration (TMR), the samples should be collected at 4 to 8 hrs after the cows get access to the fresh ration. There are following methods used for rumen liquor collection from ruminant animals:

A. Needle puncture of the rumen (rumenocentesis).

B. Oral or nasal passage of stomach tube.

C. Collection from rumen fistulated animal.

D. Collection from slaughtered animal.

A. Needle puncture of the rumen (rumenocentesis)

Rumenocentesis, the collection of rumen fluid by percutaneous needle aspiration, has become a common diagnostic test. This technique essentially involves inserting a needle into the ventral rumen and aspirating a sample of rumen fluid (Nordlund and Garrett, 1994).

Procedure

i) Landmarks for the puncture site are the left side on a horizontal line level with the top of the patella about 15 to 20 cm posterior to the last rib.

ii) The cow is restrained in a stanchion or head-lock and one assistant elevates the tail of the cow while another assistant inserts a nose leader and pulls the cow's head to the right side.

iii) A disposable needle of 4" or 5" length is thrust through the skin, then into the rumen and fluid is collected with very slight aspiration.

iv) When sufficient volume has been obtained, the air is evacuated from the syringe and pH is measured immediately.

Precaution

The needle will usually become obstructed by ingesta which is cleared by forcing a small volume of air or fluid back through the needle. When the needle becomes obstructed, it is important to avoid creating a negative pressure within the syringe as CO_2 will leave the fluid and increase the pH. Typically, 3 to 5 ml of rumen fluid can be collected with minimal difficulty.

B. Oral or nasal passage of stomach tube

Restrain the animal in a crush or head bail. The sample is collected using a stomach tube passed down the nasal passage or through the mouth. Before commencing the procedure, measure the length of tube required to be passed, to ensure that the tube will rest in the rumen.

i) Through mouth: Position a dental gag or a probang gag to allow the tube to be passed without damage from the teeth. Feed the tube gently but firmly over the base of the tongue and pass the tube into the oesophagus.

ii) Through nasal passage: Ensure that the tube is lubricated and warm before passage. Direct the tube into the ventral nasal passage and gently pass to the level of the pharynx and oesophagus. Observe for signs that the tube is present in the oesophagus and not the trachea (the beast will breathe through a tube passed into the trachea). Pass the stomach tube until it reaches the level of the rumen.

Rumen liquor collection: Attach a stirrup pump and use it to withdraw around 100 ml rumen liquor. Fluid is not always readily obtained, however adjusting the positioning of the tube may assist. When the sample is collected, kink the tube to prevent loss of ruminal fluid from the tube, and withdraw it carefully.

C. Collection from rumen fistulated animal

Collection of large volumes of rumen fluid is most easily accomplished using a rumen fistulated animal. Removal of rumen fluid is less stressful when the donor is fistulated than by stomach tubing a non-fistulated donor. The technique can be criticized on the grounds that it is an interference with the normal functioning of the animal and that if not carefully maintained the fistula and the cannula can be a source of stress.

D. Collection from slaughtered animal

About 15 minutes after slaughter, incise the middle part of the rumen of animal and scoop fresh rumen samples and filled into pre-warmed thermos flasks leaving no head space. Seal flask tightly and transport to the place of study. Transportation of rumen fluid for long distances must be done through double Jacket container.

13.2. Examination of rumen fluid

The sample should be evaluated as soon as possible after collection to minimize the effects of cooling and air exposure on protozoal activity and pH. Estimation of biochemical characters can be delayed to 9 hrs in room temperature sample and up to 24 hrs on a refrigerated sample.

Table 13.1. Physical characteristics of rumen fluid

S.No.	Characteristics		Indication
1.	Colour		
	i) Yellowish brown colour (normal)	:	Grain, silage ration, hay ration
	ii) Deeper green colour (normal)	:	Green ration
	iii) Milky gray	:	Grain overfeeding
	iv) Darker greenish	:	Prolonged ruminal stasis and/or decomposition of rumen contents.
	v) Gray with clots of milk	:	Calves with abomasal reflux or oesophegeal groove failure
2.	Consistency		
	i) Slightly viscous consistency	:	Normal
	ii) Watery	:	Inactive bacteria and protozoa
	iii) Excess frothy	:	Frothy bloat from primary tympany or vagus indigestion
3.	Odour		
	i) Aromatic acceptable odour	:	Normal
	ii) Ammonia smell	:	Urea poisoning
	iii) Moldy rotting odor (putrified)	:	Protein putrefaction

	iv) Intensely sour odor	:	Excess lactic acid production from grain or carbohydrate overfeeding
4.	pH		
	i) Ranges between 6-7 in animals on a mostly forage diet	:	Normal
	ii) Rages between 5.5-6.5 in animals fed mostly grain diet	:	Normal
	iii) Ranges between 8-10 (rumen alkalosis)	:	Simple indigestion, urea indigestion, putrefaction of rumen ingesta
	iv) Ranges between 5.0-5.5	:	Engorgement with readily digestible carbohydrates, chronic rumen acidosis, abomasal reflux from abomasal disease, vagal indigestion and intestinal obstruction

Table 13.2. Chemical characteristics of rumen fluid

S.No.	Chemical test	Indication
1.	Sedimentation activity test	Evaluation of protozoa activity
	Put a sample of rumen fluid in a test tube and let to stand. Measure the time needed for completion of sedimentation of fine particles and floatation of coarse solid particles	
	i) Prolonged time in sedimentation	Active protozoa
	ii) Very rapid sedimentation with no floatation	Rumen acidosis, prolonged anorexia, inactive microflora from indigestible roughages
	iii) No appreciable sedimentation or floatation	Frothy bloat, some cases of vagal indigestion

2.	Methylene blue reduction test	Anaerobic fermentative metabolism of the bacterial population
	Mix 20 ml of rumen fluid with 1 ml of 0.03% methylene in a test tube and let to stand at room temperature. Measure the time needed for the color of the mixture to be changed.	
	i) Decolorization within 3 minutes leaving a narrow ring of blue color at the top of decolorizing mixture	Normal fermentative activity of anaerobic bacterial
	ii) Abnormal reduction of time up to 15 minutes	Indigestible roughage, rumen acidosis
3.	Cellulose digestion test	Activity of cellulolytic bacteria
	Mix 10 ml of rumen fluid with 0.3 ml of 16 % glucose. Immerse a thread of pure cellulose. The lower end is weighted by a glass bead. Incubate the tube at 37 °C. Record the time for the bead to be dropped free at the bottom of the tube.	
	i) A fully active rumen fluid will digest the cellulose foaming within 24-30 hrs	Normal activity of cellulolytic bacteria

Table 13.3. Microscopic examination of rumen protozoa

S.No.	Microscopic examination	Indication
Examine in a fresh film under low power (X 40 to X 100) magnifying microscope		
1.	Highly motile and very crowded	+++
2.	Motile and crowded.	++
3.	Sluggish motility and low number	+
4.	No or sporadic alive protozoa	0
5.	Fauna are motile	Normal fluid
6.	Sluggish or no movement at all recent acidosis	Abnormal fluid

13.3. Ruminal bacteria counting

Rumen samples are taken by the standard methods and an aliquot of each is stored in an air tight container with a 50% formaldehyde (CH_2O) (v/v) solution in a ratio of 1:1. Preserved sample is mixed very well before bacterial counting to insure a uniform sample and free all bacteria that are bound to feed particles.

a) Procedure

i) An aliquot of 0.1 ml preserved sample is placed in a graduated cylinder and brought to 100 ml with water.

ii) Allow the particulate matter to settle out drawn on a clean sheet of paper. After cleaning with alcohol, dry a microscope slide and super impose upon the circle.

iii) With a pipette, transfer 0.01 ml of the diluted rumen fluid to the slide and center over the circle.

iv) With the 3 mm inoculum loop, transfer one loop full of the nigrosine dye solution to the slide.

v) Immediately mix the dye and the sample thoroughly with the loop. When well mixed, spread the material evenly over the entire area of the circle.

vi) Place the slide on a hot plate and dry rapidly. Once dried, the slide may be stored indefinitely.

vii) Immersion oil is placed on the slide and with great care the slide is focused on the microscope.

viii) The bacteria will appear as white spots on a dark red to black background.

ix) The slide should be observed under low power to insure that the slide is uniform. The bacteria of 50 randomly selected fields across several diameters of the slide are counted. This procedure is necessary to reduce the effect of an uneven distribution on the slide.

x) Under normal operation, the environment will add to the count. Therefore, a blank slide should be prepared with water in place of the diluted rumen material. The count of 50 fields from the blank is subtracted from the count of each sample slide.

b) Calculation

The ratio of the area of the 50 fields and the area of the circle is proportional to the ratio of the corrected number of bacteria per 50 fields and the number of organisms per sample transferred to the slide. Once, the number of bacteria transferred to the slide in 0.01 ml is known the dilution factors are used to express the count as bacteria per ml of ruminal fluid.

c) Limitations

i) The amount of dye used may need to be increased to achieve best results.

ii) It is difficult to evenly spread the material over the entire area of the circle. Therefore, a circle made with a soft wax pencil upon the slide seems to work very well.

iii) Drying should be rapid; however, this step is very sensitive and required close attention.

13.4. Ruminal protozoa counting

a) Sample collection and dilution

Ruminal contents are hand mixed as thoroughly as possible and a 50 ml plastic beaker is used to collect the sample. If hand mixing is not possible, composite samples of contents from various locations (reticulum, cranial sac, dorsal sac, and ventral sac). For counts per gram of ruminal fluid:

i) Pipette approximately 10 ml of ruminal contents with a wide mouth pipette into a tared beaker and note the weight of the sample.

ii) To the beaker, pipette 10% formalin solution with a pasteur pipette to equal the weight of ruminal contents (1:1 dilution).

iii) A 2.0 ml aliquot of the well mixed, formalinized sample is pipetted with a wide orifice pipette into a test tube containing 18 ml glycerol-buffer-methyl green mixture (1:20 final dilution).

iv) The mixture is allowed to stand for at least 4 hrs before counting, overnight results in better staining (After protozoa are fixed, stain within one week).

b) Procedure

i) Add 5 ml of ruminal fluid to 5 ml of formalin solution (dilution 1:1) and mix.

ii) Place a 2 ml aliquot of the well mixed, formalinized sample with a wide orifice pipette into a test tube containing 18 ml glycerol-buffer-methyl green mixture (1:20 final dilution).

iii) The mixture is allowed to stand for at least 4 hrs before counting, overnight results in better staining (after protozoa are fixed, stain within one week).

iv) Mix the tube well immediately before counting.

v) Fill the counting chamber (Sedgewick-Rafter Cell) and place a cover slip on the chamber carefully, without causing formation of air bubbles.

vi) The slide is set for 10 minutes to allow settling of protozoa.

vii) If dilution is too concentrated, further dilution with phosphate buffer prior to counting works well 7 to 8 protozoa per field is desirable).

viii) Use the eyepiece to count the number of organisms.

ix) Count at least 25 microscopic fields using a 10X objective.

x) It is better to count 50 fields through all the chambers.

c) Constants and calculation

1. Constant

i) Eye piece standard square units (one field)	0.469225 mm^2
ii) Depth of Sedgewick-Rafter cell	1.00 mm
iii) Standard volumetric units	0.469225 mm^3
iv) Volume of 50 field	23.461250 mm^3
v) Organisms per count (1000 mm^3/23.46125 mm^3)	46.6235

2. Calculation

Number of organisms:

50 fields x dilution x organisms per count = Organisms/ml or g

For identification of species use an atlas of microbiology. Practice the procedure before you experiment. Be consistent on time of sampling relative to feeding time.

13.5. Estimation of total volatile fatty acids

GLC technique is used for determination of VFA in rumen content. The GLC has a stationary phase, a liquid spread over the surface of a solid support. In GLC, a stream of carrier gas flows through the column. A sample is injected into the carrier gas near the head of packed chromatographic column. Separation of various components of the sample occurs as a result of multiple forces by which the column material tends to retain these components. In the gas phase the components move towards the outlet, but they are selectively retarded by the stationary phase. Consequently, all components pass through the column at varying speeds and emerge in the inverse order of their retention by the column material. Upon emerging from column the gaseous phase immediately enters a detector attached to the column. Here the individual components register a series of signals which appear as peaks on the chromatogram. The chromatographic peaks are used for qualitative and quantitative detection of the components.

a) Reagents

i) VFA solution (25 ng/ml): Transfer 2.5 g of individual VFA (acetic, propionic, butyric, valeric and iso-valeric) in separate 100 ml volumetric flask and make up the volume with distilled water.

ii) Lactic acid standard solution (100 mg/ml): Transfer 2.5 g lactic acid in a 25 ml volumetric flask and make up the volume.

iii) Pivalic acid internal standard (2.5 mg/ml): Dissolve 0.5 g pivalic acid in distilled water and dilute to 200 ml.

iv) Oxalic acid (0.12 M): Dissolve 3.782 g oxalic acid dehydrate in water and dilute to 250 ml.

v) Composite working standard: Pipette 1 ml of C_2, C_5 standard solution (reagent i), 2.5 ml lactic acid standard solution (reagent ii), 10 ml pivalic acid (reagent iii) and 25 ml oxalic acid solution (reagent iv) into a 100 ml volumetric flask and dilute to volume.

b) Procedure

i) Set the GLC according to manufacturers' instructions (e.g. gas flow: nitrogen- 24 ml/minute, hydrogen- 50 ml/minute and air- 500 ml/minute; temperature of injector- 220 °C, detector- 240 °C and oven- 175 °C).

ii) Make repeat 1.0 µl injections of the composite working standard until a stable response are obtained. The total chromatographic run time is approximately 30 minutes.

iii) Pipette 5 ml of strained rumen liquor into a 10 ml volumetric flask.

iv) Add 1 ml of the pivalic acid solution (reagent iii) and 2.5 ml of oxalic acid solution (reagent iv), then dilute to volume.

v) Centrifuge the resulting extract at 2600 g for 5 minutes.

vi) Inject 1.0 µl of the supernatant into GLC and integrate the peaks eluted.

c) Calculation

$$\text{Concentration of unknown VFA (mg / ml)} = \frac{\text{RF1}}{\text{RF2}} \times \text{standard conc.} \times 2$$

Where,

$$\text{RF1} = \frac{\text{Area of sample component peak}}{\text{Area of internal standard}}$$

$$\text{RF2} = \frac{\text{Area of known peak}}{\text{Area of internal standard}}$$

13.6. Determination of total nitrogen

When sample containing nitrogen is digested with H_2SO_4, the total nitrogen converts into ammonium sulphate $(NH_4)_2SO_4$. In the presence of alkali, ammonia is released from the ammonium sulphate and released ammonia is distilled and trapped in a known volume of standard acid, which is than back titrated with the standard alkali. The whole process is completed in three steps. The reactions during estimation are as follows (see 3.4):

A. Digestion: Organic nitrogen + Conc. H_2SO_4 = $(NH_4)_2SO_4$

B. Distillation: $(NH_4)_2SO_4 + 2NaOH = Na_2SO_4 + 2NH_3 + 2H_2O$

C. Titration: $2NH_3 + H_2SO_4 = (NH_4)_2SO_4$

A. Digestion

i) Take 5 ml strained rumen liquor in a Kjeldahl flask.

ii) Add 10 ml concentrated H_2SO_4.

iii) Add 2-3 g digestion mixture (contains K_2SO_4 and $CuSO_4$ in the ratio of 9:1).

iv) Keep the flask on digestion bench and allow gentle boiling. Bumping should be avoided.

v) When the solution becomes clear blue, then remove the flask from the digestion bench and cool it.

vi) Add 5 to 10 ml distilled water to the Kjeldahl flask. Transfer the whole material in 100 ml volumetric flask with repeated washings of distilled water. Make the volume to 100 ml.

B. Distillation

i) Set the Kjeldahl distillation assembly.

ii) Take 10 ml 0.01 N H_2SO_4 in a conical flask and add 2-3 drops of indicator.

iii) Keep the flask under the condenser in such a way that the tip of the condenser should be dipped in acid, to avoid ammonia loss during distillation.

iv) Take 10 ml aliquot of digested sample and transfer it into the Kjeldahl assembly.

v) Add 15-20 ml 40% NaOH to make the aliquot contents alkaline and put the stopper immediately.

vi) Allow distillation for 15 minutes.

C. Titration

i) Remove the flask after washing tip of the condenser with distilled water.

ii) Titrate the contents of the flask with standard 0.01 N NaOH till the pink color develops (end point).

iii) Record the volume of alkali used for titration on the burette.

iv) Run a blank using all reagents but no sample and following the whole procedure to estimate the nitrogen contents of the reagents, if any.

Calculation

1 ml 0.01 N H_2SO_4 = 0.00014 g nitrogen

$$\text{Total nitrogen (per 100 ml)} = \frac{V \times 0.00014 \times D \times 100}{v \times A}$$

Where, V = A – B, D is the dilution (volume made in volumetric flask), v is the initial volume of rumen liquor taken for the digestion, A is the aliquot taken (10 ml). Total nitrogen content is determined by subtracting values of blank with the values of sample.

13.7. Determination of trichloroacetic acid precipitable nitrogen

Trichloroacetic acid (TCA) precipitable nitrogen is the nitrogen coming from the true protein because by adding trichloroacetic acid, only proteins are precipitated. These precipitated proteins are analyzed further for nitrogen contents by Micro Kjeldahl method.

A. Procedure

i) Take 5.0 ml rumen liquor in a centrifuge tube.

ii) Add 5.0 ml of 20% TCA.

iii) Leave the tubes overnight.

iv) Centrifuge the tubes at 2,000 rpm for 10 minutes.

v) Transfer the whole precipitate with repeated washings of distilled water in Kjeldahl flask.

vi) Proceed for digestion, distillation and titration as described above (see 10.6).

13.8. Determination of soluble nitrogen

Soluble nitrogen = Total nitrogen - TCA precipitable nitrogen

13.9. Determination of ammonia nitrogen

In alkaline medium, ammonia is released from the rumen liquor and the released ammonia is analyzed for nitrogen contents by Micro-Kjeldahl method.

Procedure: Take 5.0 ml strained rumen liquor in the distillation assembly and 5 ml of 40% NaOH. Proceed for distillation and titration as described above (see 10.6).

13.10. Determination of lactic acid

Lactic acid, when heated with concentrated H_2SO_4, converts into acetaldehyde, which reacts with p-hydroxydiphenyl to give purple color in the presence of copper ions.

a) Reagents

i) Copper sulphate (20%): Dissolve 200 g $CuSO_4.5H_2O$ in 500 ml distilled water and make the volume to one litre. The solution is stable indefinitely.

ii) Copper sulphate (4%): Take 200 ml of reagent 1, and make the volume to one litre.

iii) Calcium hydroxide.

iv) Concentrated sulphuric acid.

v) NaOH (5%): 5 g NaOH, dissolve in 100 ml distilled water.

vi) p-hydroxydiphenyl reagent: Take 1.5 g p-dyroxydiphenyl in a 100 ml volumetric flask. Add 100 ml of 5% NaOH and 100 ml distilled water. Warm it with constant stirring to dissolve. Make the volume to 100 ml. Store it in amber color bottle.

vii) Stock standard lactic acid: Take 0.1065 g lithium lactate in 100 ml volumetric flask and dissolve in about 50 ml distilled water. Add 0.1 ml concentrated H_2SO_4 and make up the volume to 100 ml with distilled water. The solution contains 1 mg lactic acid per ml and the solution is stable for a long period in refrigerator.

viii) Working standard lactic acid solution: Dilute 1 ml of stock lactic acid solution to 100 ml with distilled water. It contains 0.01 mg lactic acid per ml. Prepare fresh working solution at the time of analysis.

b) Procedure

i) Take 1 ml strained rumen liquor in a centrifuge tube. Add 1 ml of 20% $CuSO_4$ make the volume to 10 ml.

ii) Add 1 g $Ca(OH)_2$, shake vigorously to make the mixture homogenous.

iii) Leave the tubes for 90 minutes with periodic shaking.

iv) Centrifuge at 3000 rpm for 10 minutes.

v) Take 1 ml supernatant in a test tube in duplicate.

vi) Add 0.05 ml of 4% $CuSO_4$.

vii) Add 6ml concentrated H_2SO_4 drop by drop with continuous shaking.

❑❑❑

14

Assessment of Nutritional Quality of Silage

14.1. Sampling 113

14.2. Silage quality assessment 114

14.3. Determination of silage pH 115

14.4. Determination of ammonia nitrogen 115

14.5. Determination of volatile fatty acids 116

14.6. Determination of lactic acid 117

Ensiling is a forage preservation method based on spontaneous lactic acid fermentation under anaerobic conditions. Silage techniques minimize the loss of nutrients right from harvest, to storage. The epiphytic (existing on plants) lactic acid bacteria that are present on forage crops are involved in the fermentation water-soluble carbohydrates to lactic acid and, to a lesser extent, to acetic acid. As a result the pH level of the ensiled material is reduced so the activity of spoilage microorganisms is inhibited.

14.1. Sampling

To help ensure representative samples are taken, the following key procedures are recommended:

1. Representative samples should be made by taking 1 to 5 kg of silage from different locations of the freshly open front silo. Avoid taking samples from the periphery of the silo and from moldy or damaged parts.
2. Samples should be thoroughly mixed and if the final sample has to be reduced before being sent to the laboratory, it should be prepared by the quartering method outlined below:

i) Tip the sample onto a clean surface such as a clean board or worktop. Rough concrete is not suitable.

ii) Thoroughly mix the sample ensuring an even distribution of material.

iii) Using a clean board or card, halve the sample by dividing across the pile and separating into two piles. If one pile is approximately 1 kg, carefully place this into a clean plastic bag ensuring all the material in the pile is included.

iv) After placing in the plastic bag, remove as much of the air as possible by squeezing the bag, and seal. This will help reduce silage changes during transport and make your analysis more accurate.

v) Label the bag clearly with sample number, forage mixture, stage of maturity and date harvested, and store immediately in a cold place, preferably in a freezer to prevent bacterial decay, until analyzed.

14.2. Silage quality assessment

Silage can either evaluated for quality by assessment of fermentation quality or by conventional feed analysis. The quality assessment by conventional feed analysis has similarities to the general methodology of feed analysis procedures already described. Focus will be made on fermentation quality assessment. Special mention is made for dry matter that needs to be corrected for volatile components including ammonia and volatile organic acids.

Extraction of silage juice: Silage "juice" extraction is made on fresh or frozen samples. Frozen samples should be kept in tight bags and left in room temperature (15-20 °C) overnight. Juice may be extract by pressing or maceration. Maceration is recommended because pressing is not applicable for silages with high DM contents. The following procedure is recommended:

i) 200 g of wet silage sample are weighed in a 1 l beaker to which add 1 l of de-ionized water. Mix carefully and leave overnight at 4 °C.

ii) Blend the sample for 2 minutes and filter through coarse (20–25 µm pore size) filter paper.

The extract will be used to determine pH, ammonia, volatile fatty acids (acetic, propionic, butyric and iso–butyric acids) and lactic acid.

14.3. Determination of silage pH

The pH is a key criteria to evaluate silage fermentation. Generally, the lower the pH, the better preserved and more stable is the silage. Haylage should reach a final pH of around 4.5 and corn silage near 4.0. The pH of the forage alone is not a good indicator of the quality of the silage, or the type of fermentation that occurred. Forages ensiled at moisture levels greater than 70% may develop large populations of clostridia bacteria, which produce butyric acid rather than lactic acid. This may result in sour silage with a pH of 5.0 or above. pH is measured directly using a conventional digital pH meter.

14.4. Determination of ammonia nitrogen

Ammonia nitrogen (NH_3-N) shows the proportion of N that has been broken down during ensilage and is the best indicator of silage fermentation. A value less than 50 g/kg N indicates an excellent fermentation, a stable silage and minimal nutrient loss. Values more than 150 g/kg N indicate a poor fermentation (Weatherburn, 1967).

a) Reagents or solutions

i) Solution A: contains, 10 g/l phenol and 0.05 g/l sodium nitroprusside with Fe^{3+}.

ii) Solution B: contains, 5 g/l NaOH and 8.4 ml/l NaClO.

iii) Preparation of ammonia solution (100 µg NH_4/ml): Dry the $(NH_4)_2SO_4$ at 105 °C in an oven for 1 hr. Dissolve 4.714 g of the previous dry reagent in 1000 ml of distilled water. Using the basic solution of ammonia, prepare a solution containing 10 µg of NH_3–N/ml (add 99 ml of water to 1 ml of the basic solution of ammonia). Prepare a standard curve using the previous solution (10 µg $(NH_4)_2SO_4$ /ml), as follows : put 0, 1, 2, 4, 6, 8 and 10 ml of the solution in 7 test tubes, adjusting the volume to 10 ml with distilled water. Stir the tubes.

b) Silage extract conditioning

i) Pipette 5 ml of the silage extract in a centrifugation tube, keeping it cold on ice.

ii) Centrifuge at 4000 rpm for 20 minutes at 4 °C.

iii) Take 0.1 ml from the supernatant and add 4.9 ml of distilled water. Stir and keep cold on ice.

c) Procedure

i) Take 1 ml of each tube from the standard curve and the unknowns.

ii) Add 5 ml of solution A and stir.

iii) Add 5 ml of solution B and stir (up to this step, keep the samples on ice).

iv) Prepare a blank containing 1 ml water, 5 ml of solution A and 5 ml of solution B.

v) Incubate at 37 °C for 20 minutes. Optionally, keep at 20 °C or more, for at least 30 minutes.

vi) Read absorbance at 625 nm.

vii) Make a standard curve using the concentrations of NH_3-N in µg/ml as abscissas and the optical density as the ordinates.

d) Calculation

From the calibration curve, calculate the concentration of the unknown samples, by interpolation. The ratio NH_3-N /total nitrogen is used as indicator of the fermentation quality.

14.5. Determination of volatile fatty acids

a) Sample preparation (Jouany, 1981)

The silage juice should be stabilized immediately. For this purpose the following steps are recommended:

i) Preparation of a conservation reagent: a solution is prepared by adding ortho H_3PO_4 (5 % v/v) and $HgCl_2$ (1 % w/v).

ii) To 10 ml of silage juice add 1 ml of the conservation reagent.

iii) Store at –15 °C in a deep freezer.

iv) Prior to analysis, fresh or frozen samples are centrifuged at 2000 rpm for 5 minutes at 4 °C.

b) Chromatography

GC equipped with flame ionization detector is used to determine VFA content in silage extract. The analysis is conducted by injecting 1 ml sample (including the conservation reagent) to which is added 0.1 ml of internal standard composed of 1% (w/v) 4-methyl valeric acid.

Calculation

VFA analysis is based on a standard solution (solution A) and an internal standard, which help determine the "response factor" used for calculation.

14.6. Determination of lactic acid

Lactic acid gives an indication of the quality of forage fermentation, being produced almost exclusively by the lactobacilli responsible for good silage fermentation and effective preservation. Higher values suggesting more rapid fermentation, better protein preservation and less likelihood of fermentation of by-products that reduces intake. Some common reasons for low lactic acid content are as follows:

i) Restricted fermentation due to high DM content (especially legumes and grasses with more than 50% DM).

ii) Restricted fermentation due to cold weather.

iii) Sample taken after considerable aerobic exposure that has degraded lactic acid.

iv) Silages high in butyric acid (clostridial silages) are usually low in lactic acid.

a) Procedure

The method suggested uses a simple colorimetric assay based on the method developed by Barker and Summerson (1941), and modified by Taylor in 1996. In this method, acetaldehyde is released from lactic acid by hot sulfuric acid. The acetaldehyde is reacted with copper and p-phenylphenol (pPP) to yield a chromagen, which absorbs at 570 nm. To develop a lactic acid standard curve:

i) Add 0 to 30 μg of lactic acid to 16 × 150 mm borosilicate tubes. The curve should be in 5 μg increments or less.

ii) Add 3 ml of concentrated H_2SO_4 and mix with a vortex mixer. This quantity of acid is defined here as 82% acid.

iii) Incubate at 95–100 °C for 10 minutes in a steam water bath.

iv) Cool at room temperature using a water bath.

v) Add 50 μl $CuSO_4$ (4%) reagent and then 100 μl of pPP reagent (1.5% p-phenylphenol in 95% ethanol); mix well on vortex mixer keeping the tube at room temperature.

vi) Leave the tubes at room temperature for at least 30 minutes and then read absorbance at 570 nm.

vii) Blanks will show values of 0.2–0.5 compared to water.

The typical assay involved 1 ml of silage juice sample to which reagents and procedures described above for the standard curve are applied. Absorbance obtained is plotted against the standard curve to calculate the amount of lactic acid.

□□□

15

Detection of Adulterants in Animal Feed

15.1. Adulteration or contamination evaluation methods . 119

15.2. Physical evaluation 119

15.3. Chemical evaluation 123

15.4. Biological evaluation 129

Adulteration is defined as the admixture of a pure substance with some cheaper and low quality substance. It is done intentionally usually to make money. Quality control is defined as the maintenance of quality at levels and tolerances acceptable to the buyer while minimizing the cost of processing. The objective of quality control of feedstuffs is to ensure that a consumer should obtain feeds that are unadulterated, true to their nature and produce desired results. Quality control in India is regulated by Bureau of Indian Standards (BIS; established under BIS Act, 1986). Earlier, Indian Standards Institute was regulating the quality control of various feed commodities.

15.1. Adulteration or contamination evaluation methods

The feedstuffs are usually evaluated by following methods:

A. Physical evaluation

B. Chemical evaluation

C. Biological evaluation

15.2. Physical evaluation

Physical evaluation is easy but less accurate in nature. One must be highly trained to identify the changes in the nature of the raw material (Chandrasekaran Natarajan and Sundram, 2001).

Table 15.1. Confirmation of feeds by physical evaluation

S.No.	Physical evaluation	Confirmation
1.	Colour	Any change in the colour of the feed ingredients gives an indication of the maturity of the grain, storage condition, presence of toxins, contamination, and possible use of insecticides/ fungicides which gives dull and dusty appearance. Orange to red colour of sorghum indicates high tannin content. Browning or blackening due to heat on improper storage reduces nutritive value. Black colour fish meal indicates the rancidity of fish fat.
2.	Size	Size of the grains governs its nutritional value due to the proportional decrease/increase in seed and its coat. Smaller the grain lower will be the metabolizable energy (ME) value due to more proportion of coater hulls. Higher weight indicates a higher ME value.
3.	Smell	Smell is the next best indicator just standing near the stock itself will immediately indicate any difference in the normal smell. Any change in the normal smell of the ingredients should be viewed with suspicion. Musty odour indicates the beginning of fungal contamination or boring insects. To detect rancidity in oil rich feed ingredients this is the best method. Odour of petroleum products is suggestive of excessive pesticides or fungicides. Leathery smell of meat meal indicates its adulteration with leather meal.
4.	Taste	Each ingredient has a different taste, any change in the taste like bitterness in the grains, soya, sunflower oil meal and groundnut cake indicates the presence of mycotoxins. The level of salt can be detected by tasting the ingredient and the feed. Bitter taste of rice polish indicates the rancidity of the fatty acids.
5.	Homogeneity	The presence of contaminants like other grains, husk, broken grains, weed seeds, infested seeds is viewed. In the oil seed cakes closer

		observation will reveal the presence of fibrous material, especially in de-oiled groundnut cake, the cake with hulls which contains nearly 20-30% crude fibre can be visually identified.
6.	Touch	Feeling the raw material will indicate the dryness. Chillness indicates high moisture content. Clumps can be found out by inserting the hand inside the bag. The clumps may be due to high moisture content, improper storage, and packaging of fresh warm solvent extracted meal. Clumps formed due to excess of moisture will be very hard.
7.	Sound	Dry grains on pouring down or biting will produce sound of spilling coins.

Feed microscopy

Feed microscopy is commonly used for confirming the adulteration and identifying the adulterants. Feed ingredients, adulterants and contaminants must be studied under low and high magnification for distinguishing features whether coarsely or finely ground. At physical characteristics such as shape, colour, and particle size, softness, hardness, and texture of the feeds are examined at low magnification of 8X to 50X. The plant cells and structural features of the feeds are observed at high magnification of 100X to 500X since their characters are retained after grinding or even after powdering the feed ingredients. A feed scientist must be familiar with of feed ingredients and adulterants and must have a collection of pure feed ingredients, adulterants and contaminants for the accurate and fast quality assurance results.

Table 15.2. Precise characteristics on microscopic identification (Khajaren *et al.*, 1987)

S.No.	Identification	Confirmation
1	Yellow to brown oval helium with a clear slit, pox-marked outer surface hull, hourglass and palisade cells from the hull are the major cellular keys for soybeans and also elongated cells below the peripheral cells of the cotyledon	Soybean meal
2	Thin skin with copper to red colour, highly pitted cell of pod fragment and the lack of palisade cells in the testa, elongated pit in hypodermal stone cells and unique cross fibre cell of pod.	Groundnut meal
3	The inner surface seed coat has a delicate semi transparent white sheet adhering to the surface	Rapeseed meal/ mustard oil cake
4	Long flat and twisted fibre adhering to the hulls, kernel fragments are yellow to brown containing many round, red, brown gossypol glands. The hull edge has a light brown layer with stairstep facets. The epidermal cells are heavy walled with dark pigmented interiors. Palisade cells can also be used for identification.	Cottonseed meal
5	Striped or all black varieties for the hull, leathery hull with a paper-like lining. Twin hairs, united almost to their tips on the outer surface of the cypsela unbroken pericarp fragment may appear as broken pieces in the medium, the outer epiderm of transversely elongated cells with zigzag walls	Sunflower meal
6	Seed coat or outer epidermal cells contain calcium oxalate crystals with black brown or yellow brown coloured and granular surface.	Sesame meal
7	Curved scales with concentric rays, bone exhibit lacunae with well defined	Fish meal

	canaliculi, milky glass beads with broken surface eye lenses	
8	Spherical particle, smooth surface with glass when rubbed dark red to almost black in colour	Blood meal

15.3. Chemical evaluation

Proximate analysis and chemical tests are generally used as chemical evaluates.

A. Proximate analysis

Analysis of feedstuffs for proximate principles provides preliminary information about nutrient composition. Proximate analysis is still the most widely used feed analysis methods, although some other methods are available. Low CP and high CF of oil seed meals are indicative of adulteration with fibrous material. The high CP alone is indicative of adulteration with urea and or some inferior quality oil seed meals like mahua, castor or karanja cake. The amount of AIA is a good guide to the amount of sand or other which may be present. The fish meals are usually adulterated with sand during drying process.

B. Chemical tests for adulteration determination

Diverse spot and laboratory chemical tests are available for determination of quality and adulteration in feed. Some common tests are as follows (Khajaren and Khajaren, 1998).

1. Salt in fish meal

Very high amount of salt (NaCl), present especially in jawala fish, can cause problem when added in poultry rations. Salt in fish meal (more than 4%) cause many abnormalities in the birds e.g. diarrhoea, salt poisoning etc.

Procedure

Chloride ions, present as potassium chloride, are detected by treating the water extract of feed sample with standard silver nitrate. The intensity of brick red precipitate formed indicates the presence of salt in the sample.

i) Transfer about 2 g ground sample in a beaker and add 90 ml hot water.

ii) Stir it with a glass rod. Keep it aside for 5 to 10 minutes.

iii) Filter the extract through muslin cloth.

iv) Take 10 ml filtrate in a beaker and add 3 to 4 drops saturated potassium chromate solution as an indicator.

v) Add drop wise 0.1 N silver nitrate with a dropper in to the beaker.

Confirmation: Formation of brick red colour precipitate indicates the presence of chloride in the sample. Higher the concentration of brick red colour precipitate, more the salt in the sample.

2. Urea in protein rich feed

Urea is one of the NPN source and cannot be used for feeding of monogastric animals. Certain protein rich poultry feed ingredients like fish meal; ground nut cake etc. may be adulterated by urea to increase the total nitrogen content.

Procedure

Urea in feed and feed ingredients is extracted by treating with zinc acetate in glacial acetic acid (Carrez solution 1) and potassium ferrocyanide (Carrez solution 2). When the filtrate is treated with dimethylaminobenzaldehyde (DMAB) reagents, the intensity of yellow colour which develops is directly proportional to the concentration of urea.

i) Take 1 g finely ground sample into a 500 ml volumetric flask.

ii) Add 1 g activated charcoal, 250 ml Carrez solution 1 and 5 ml Carrez solution 2.

iii) Shake and dilute it to 500 ml water and keep it for half an hr.

iv) Take 5 ml filtrate in a test tube and add 5 ml DMAB solution into it and shake.

Confirmation: The yellow colour intensity will directly reflect the amount of urea present in the test tube.

3. Evaluation of mahua cake adulteration

The method is based on the principle that the saponin gives a typical colour test when extracted and reacted with antimony trichloride.

Procedure

i) Take 10 g of the finely ground material in the extraction thimble.

ii) Tap it to pack it well and pour rectified spirit into the tube so as to soak the sample.

iii) Collect the first drop of extract on a Whatman filter paper 1 (10 cm diameters).

iv) Dry and then wash it with 2 to 3 drops of distilled water in the centre of the dried spot.

v) Dry the filter paper completely.

vi) Dip the paper in a beaker containing antimony trichloride solution and dry it on a spirit lamp or a burner. Care should be taken not to overheat the paper which will be evident by its charring.

Confirmation: Appearance of a pink colour after heating for 5 minutes indicates the presence of mahua cake.

4. Detection of castor husk or castor cake

The method is based on the fact that castor husk is not bleached under the conditions which cause the bleaching of almost all other materials of vegetable origin likely to be present in an oil cake. The method consists of the treatment of the material with dilute alkali and acid solutions followed by treatment with bleaching powder solution and isolation of the unbleached castor husk.

Procedure

i) Take three separate 100 g portion of the feed material and boil for 30 minutes with 1 l of sodium hydroxide solution (5%).

ii) Filter through muslin cloth, boil again for 30 minutes with one litre of hydrochloric acid solution (5%) and filter.

iii) Digest the residue for a period depending upon the type of the oil cake, with the solution of bleaching powder (5%).

iv) When bleaching is complete, filter off the solution, spread the bleached residue in a thin layer, under water in a white photographic tray.

v) Remove any black pieces and examine microscopically. After identification, compare the pieces with portion of castor husk, which have also undergone the above treatment (control).

Confirmation: Castor husk has a distinctive pitted surface, when examined in reflected light under a microscope.

Other method used for detection of ricin is injection of ricin in immunized rabbit. The ricin is extracted from 10 g feed and injected to immunized rabbit and mortality is observed. The immune serum will not prevent death from any substance other than ricin. Injecting the extract of a feedstuff (containing castor cake) mixed with normal serum causes greater mortality in rabbit. This test can detect 1 ppm of ricin.

Another method of detecting castor cake is the used potassium chlorate. When feed is treated with potassium chlorate, the castor cake is destroyed and settles down at the bottom.

5. Detection of neem seed cake adulteration

The coarsely grounded feed is extracted in 95% alcohol at room temperature. Extract is concentrated under room reduce pressure till a thick syrup amber colour residue is obtained which is treated with different solvents to extract a crystalline product (Nimbin). It is continuously dissolved in concentrate sulphuric acid, the brown solution changes to cherry red on addition of small quantity of concentrated nitric acid. The crystalline product gives a yellow colour with tetranitromethane. A alcoholic solution of the crystalline product shows a sky blue florescence under ultraviolet light.

6. Detection of linseed meal in animal feed

Small amount of feed is treated with 1-2 drops of diluted H_2SO_4 acid in a micro test tube. The mouth of the test tube is covered with a disk of filter paper moisten with a drop of reagent. Depending upon the amount of HCN produced a more or less intense blue appearance on the reagent paper confirms the presence of linseed meal in feed. Gentle warming in water bath is advisable when small quantity of cyanide is suspected.

7. Detection of cotton seed cake in animal feed

Weight about 200 mg of feed sample into screw cap in test tubes and extract cycloprenoids and then measure it colorimetrically.

8. Measurement of quality of soybean meal

Quality of soybean meal is tested for the presence of trypsin inhibitors and haemagglutinins, which depress the utilization proteins and for urease activity, an indicator of level of cooking or processing applied during the preparation of soybean meal. Spread the sample uniformly on petri dish, glazed paper with white background. Visual examination of soybean meal when treated with urea-phenol red solution (dissolve 0.14 g of phenol red in 7 ml 0.1 N NaOH and 35 ml distilled water. Dissolve 21 g of urea in 300 ml distilled water. Mixed these two solutions together and titrate to amber colour with 0.1 N H_2SO_4).

Table 15.3. Visual examination of soybean meal when treated with urea-phenol red solution

S.No.	Appearance	Urease activity	Urease content	Assessment
1	No red colour particles	Inactive	0.00	Overcooked
2	Few scattered red particles	Slightly active	0.05-0.10	Properly cooked
3	Approximately 25% red particles	Moderately active	0.20	Properly cooked
4	Approximately 50% or more red particles	Very active	Above 0.20 cooked	Under

9. Detection of horn and hoof in animal feed

Take 2 to 3 particles of amber colour test sample into an evaporating dish and add 5 ml of glacial acetic acid into the evaporating dish and let stand for 60 minutes. If hoof and horn are present, the test particles will still hard and tough. Gelatin will become soft and swollen.

10. Detection of leather meal in animal feed

Select brown to black test sample particles and place in petri dish and add 3 to 5 drops of ammonium molybdate and let it stand for

5 to 10 minutes. Leather meal will give no colour change. Meat and bone meal gives a greenish yellow colour.

11. Detection of plant protein and animal protein in animal feed

Carbohydrates from plant contain starch and cellulose. When it react with iodine and chlor-zinc iodine solution, the starchy tissue releases a blue colour and cellulose develops a purple colour when examine under a microscope.

i) Extract 1 to 2 g of test sample in 100 ml boiling water for 2 to 3 minutes.

ii) Take 3 to 5 ml of cool extract in test tube and add 5 to 6 drops of iodine solution.

iii) If starch is present, the mixture turns blue.

iv) Spread 1 to 2 g of test sample into a petri plate and add 5 to 6 drops of chlor-zinc iodine solution and let stand for 10 minutes.

v) A purple brown colour indicated the presence of plant fibre (cellulose), whereas yellow indicated animal fibre (protein) using a microscopic examination.

12. Detection of heavy metals in animal feed

Extract 1 to 2 g of the test material into 10 ml distilled water. Then take 3 drops each of ammonium carbonate (10%), ammonium sulfide (20%) and potassium iodide (1%) reagents at different places on a marble slab. Put two drops of metal solution over these spots. Mix them properly and observe the colour formed. Match it with the chart and detect the metal.

Table 15.4. Visual examination of presence of heavy metals in animal feed

S.No.	Metal	Test solutions		
		Ammonium carbonate	**Ammonium sulfide**	**Potassium iodide**
1.	Antimony	White	Orange	No reaction
2.	Arsenic	No reaction	Yellow	No reaction
3.	Barium	White	No reaction	No reaction
4.	Bismuth	White	Brown	Brown
5.	Copper	Light blue	Black	Brown
6.	Lead	White	Black	Golden yellow
7.	Mercury	White	Black	Green terns to red
8.	Zinc	White	White	No reaction

15.4. Biological evaluation

Biological evaluation of the feed involves the use of animals, specialized persons to conduct the digestion and metabolism trials on the various species of livestock and poultry. The detail about digestion and metabolism trials are depicted in chapter number 11. Another example of biological evaluation of feeds is the extraction of ricin from 10 g feed with different solvents present in castor cake and injected into immunized rabbit and mortality is observed. The immune serum will not prevent death from any substance other than ricin. Injecting the extract of a feedstuffs (containing castor cake) mixed with normal serum causes greater mortality in rabbits and rodents.

❑❑❑

16

Detection of Anti-Nutritional Factors in Feed

16.1. Determination of protease inhibitors 133
16.2. Tannin determination 139
16.3. Methods for nitrates and nitrites analysis 146
16.4. Determination of hydrocyanic acid 148
16.5. Determination of total oxalate contents 150
16.6. Determination of saponin 152
16.7. Gossypol determination 153
16.8. Determination of mycotoxin 155

Anti-nutritional factors (ANFs) are substances that when present in animal feed or water they either by themselves or through their metabolic products reduce the availability of one or more nutrients. The ANFs may be classified on the basis of their effects on the nutritional value of feedstuffs, and on the biological response to them in the animal.

Table 16.1. Common anti-nutritional factors present in animal feeds and fodders

S.No.	Anti-nutritional factor	Adverse effect	Source
1.	Protease inhibitor	Inhibits activity of trypsin and chymotrypsin enzymes. Interferes with the availability of methionine amino acid	Soybean, kidney bean, mung bean and other legume seeds
2.	Haemagglutinins	Agglutination of the RBC	Soybean, castor bean and other legume seeds
3.	Saponins	Foaming property in aqueous solution (bloat/ tympany), haemolyse RBC	Lucerne and soybean forages
4.	Cyanogens	Excess HCN can quickly produce anoxia of the central nervous system inactivating the cytochrome oxidase	Jowar, linseed, other mature fodder and grasses etc
5.	Glucosinolates	Interferes with the availability of iodine (goitrogenic)	Brassica genus
6.	Gossypol	Interferes with the availability of iron (olive green colour egg yolk)	Gossypium genus
7.	Tannins	Tannins bind the proteins and are thus inhibitors of Proteolytic enzymes (depress protein digestibility)	Sorghum, Salseed meal, Mangoseed kernel etc
8.	Phytic acid	Depresses the utilization of several minerals such as Ca, Mg, Fe, Zn, etc	Wheat, maize, rice, barley, oat, soybean etc
9.	Oxalic acid	Interferes with the availability of Ca	Depress growth and blood Ca level
10.	Anti-vitamin K	Sweet clover disease or bleeding disease in cattle	Sweet clover

16.1. Determination of protease inhibitors

Activities of these inhibitors represented as trypsin inhibitor activity (TIA) values. TIA can be measured by the use of following methods:

A. Quantification of trypsin inhibitory activity using azocasein

B. Quantification of trypsin inhibitory activity using benzoyl-L-arginine-p-ni- troanilide (L-BAPA)

C. Quantification of trypsin inhibitory activity using bromocresol purple index (BCPI)

A. Quantification of trypsin inhibitory activity using azocasein (Spelbrink *et al.*, 2011)

Procedure

i) Prepare a 30 g/l azocasein stock solution by dissolving the protein in 100 mM pH 8.5 Tris-buffer containing 5 mM of $CaCl_2$ at 50 °C and cooling back to 37 °C.

ii) Accurately weigh trypsin for a concentration between 0.3 and 0.4 mg/ml and dissolve in 1 mM HCl solution. Prepare trypsin solution immediately prior to analysis.

iii) Disperse sample material in pH 3.3 acetic acid solution.

iv) From the sample material, prepare a series of dilutions in such a way as cause a 50% loss of signal upon incubation for the highest sample concentration.

v) From each dilution, mix 125 µl with 25 µl of trypsin stock solution in an eppendorf cup, or with 25 µl of demineralised water as a control. Use 125 µl of demineralised water rather than sample material for positive and negative controls.

vi) To these mixtures, add 225 µl of warm azocasein followed by 30 minutes incubation at 37 °C.

vii) The reaction is then quenched by the addition of 150 µl of 15% (w/v) TCA solution. The order of addition of azocasein is the same as the order of addition of TCA to ensure equal incubation times for all samples.

viii) Non-hydrolysed azocasein and other insoluble are remove by centrifugation at 15,000 g at 4 °C for 10 minutes.

ix) Transfer 100 μl of the supernatants to a microtiter plate by careful pipetting and supplement with 100 μl of 1.5 M NaOH solution. The plate is then analysing for absorbance at 450 nm on a microplate reader.

Calculation

The absorbances are plotted against the amount of sample material in the plate. The slope of the resulting line is obtained *via* linear regression using the least squares method and indicates the amount of absorbance lost per quantity of sample material. The positive control, in the absence of sample, indicates the maximum absorbance cause by the known quantity of trypsin. Hence, by dividing the slope by the positive controls' absorbance, the TIA express as the amount of trypsin inhibited per amount of sample material is obtain.

B. Quantification of trypsin inhibitory activity using L-BAPA (ISO14902:2001)

The determination of trypsin inhibitor activity can be perform by using the ISO specifies method. This trypsin inhibitor activity is indicative of the degree of toasting of these products. The detection limit of the method is 0.5 mg/g. Principle of TIA is based on extraction of trypsin inhibitors from the sample at pH 9.5. The remaining trypsin activity is measured by adding benzoyl-L-arginine-p-nitroanilide (L-BAPA) as substrate. The quantity of released p-nitroaniline is measured spectrometrically.

Reagents

0.01 mol/l NaOH, 0.001, 0.1, 1 and 6 mol/l HCH, 5.3 mol/l CH_3COOH, $CaCl_2.2H_2O$, Calcium chloride solution in hydrochloric acid (dissolves 735 mg of calcium chloride dihydrate in 1 l of hydrochloric acid and adjust pH to 3.0), bovine trypsin, trypsin stock solution (allow the trypsin to reach room temperature. Dissolve 27 mg of trypsin in the calcium chloride solution in a 100 ml volumetric flask and dilute to the mark with the calcium chloride solution. This solution can be used for 5 days at most when stored in the refrigerator), trypsin working solution (pipette 5 ml of the trypsin stock solution into a 100 ml volumetric flask and dilute to the mark with calcium chloride solution), L-BAPA, tris-(hydroxymethyl) aminomethane (tris), dimethyl sulfoxide (DMSO), tris buffer/caicium chloride solution (dissolve 6.05 g of Tris and 735 mg of calcium chloride in 900 ml of water in a 1 l graduated measuring cylinder. Adjust the pH to 8.2 with hydrochloric acid and dilute to 1 l with water), L-BAPA reagent (prepare this reagent on the day of use. Dissolve 60 mg of L-BAPA in 1 ml of DMSO in a 100 ml volumetric flask and dilute to the mark with Tris buffer/calcium chloride solution).

Procedure

i) Weigh 1 g of the ground and thoroughly mix test sample in a 100 ml conical flask and add 50 ml of 0.01 mol/l NaOH solution. Completely suspend the sample.

ii) Adjust the pH to 9.5 with hydrochloric acid (1 and 0.1 mol/l). Rinse the electrode with as little distilled water as possible.

iii) Close the conical flask and store overnight in the refrigerator (4 °C). Place in the refrigerator the quantity of water needed for making up the sample extracts.

iv) Transfer the sample extract to a 100 ml volumetric flask.

v) Dilute to the mark with distilled water from the refrigerator and mix. Store the volumetric flask in the refrigerator. The sample extract remains stable for one day. After sedimentation for 15 minutes, the sample extract may be worked up further and diluted as required. Dilutions depend on the expected TIA value of the sample and are carried out with water at room temperature.

vi) Estimate the TIA value of the sample and prepare three different dilutions of the sample extract on the basis of the dilution scheme so that it may be expected that as a result of the TIA measurement at least one of the three inhibition percentages obtained will be within the range of 40-60%.

Dilution scheme

Attributes	Blank standard (ml)	Standard (ml)
Pipette into centrifuge tubes according to the following scheme:		
L-BAPA reagent	5	5
Distilled water	3	3
Acetic acid (5.3 mol/l)	1	0
Mix the contents of the tubes with the test tube mixer (6.5) and place the tubes in the water bath (37 °C) for 10 minutes and add		
Trypsin working solution	1	1
Mix the contents of the tubes with the test tube mixer and place the centrifuge tubes back in the water bath. After 10 minutes of incubation, add the following:		
Acetic acid (5.3 mol/l)	0	1

vii) Mix the contents of the tubes with the test tube mixer.

viii) Centrifuge the tubes for 10 minutes in the centrifuge at a radial acceleration of approximately 1500 g.

ix) Measure the absorbance of the clear solutions relative to water in the spectrometer at 410 nm. These solutions remain stable for at least 2 hrs.

Measurement of trypsin activity

i) For determination of trypsin activity in working solution, the difference between the absorbance of the working solution and the absorbance of the blank (Ar - Abr) should be 0.380. If this is not the case, check the quality of the trypsin.

ii) For determination of trypsin activity in sample, prepare each dilution of sample extract a corresponding blank solution. Sample extract solution and corresponding blank solutions shall be dealt with simultaneously in the procedure, including centrifuging.

Dilution scheme

Attributes	Blank standard (ml)	Standard (ml)	Blank sample (ml)	Sample (ml)
L-BAPA reagent	5	5	5	5
Diluted sample extract	0	0	1	1
Distilled water	3	3	2	2
Acetic acid (5.3 mol/l)	1	0	1	0
Mix the contents of the tubes with the test tube mixer and place the tubes in the water bath (37 °C) for 10 minutes. Add the following:				
Trypsin working solution	1	1	1	1
Mix the contents of the tubes with the test tube mixer and place the centrifuge tubes back in the water bath (37 °C). After 10 minutes incubation add the following:				
Acetic acid (5.3 mol/l)	0	1	0	1

iii) Mix the contents of the tubes with the test tube mixer.

iv) Centrifuge the tubes for 10 minutes in the centrifuge at a radial acceleration of approximately 1500 g.

v) Measure the absorbance of the clear solutions relative to water in the spectrometer at 410 nm. These solutions remain stable for at least 2 hrs.

Calculation

i) Calculate the inhibition percentage of the sample extract solutions by the equation:

$$i = \frac{(Ar - Abr) - (As - Abs)}{(Ar - Abr)} \times 100\%$$

Where, i is the inhibition percentage, Ar is the absorbance of the solution with standard, Abr is the absorbance of the blank with standard, As is the absorbance of the solution with sample and Abs is the absorbance of the blank with sample.

ii) Calculate the trypsin inhibitor activity, expressed in milligrams of inhibited trypsin per gram of sample, by the equation:

$$TIA = \frac{i}{100\%} \times \frac{ml\ f1\ f2}{mo}$$

Where, TIA is the trypsin inhibitor activity, in milligrams per gram, i is the inhibition percentage, in percent, mo is the mass of the test sample, in grams, m1 is the mass of trypsin, in milligrams, f1 is the dilution of the sample extract [(100 ml x 100 ml)/V], where V is the volume and f2 is a conversion factor (2.8×10^{-4}) based on the purity of trypsin (56 %).

C. Quantification of trypsin inhibitory activity using bromocresole purple index (BCPI)

Analyses using bromocresole purple index method (BCPI) is perform according to the procedure postulated by Szmigielski (2004).

Procedure

i) This analytical procedure involve: grinding of the representative sample and sieving them through 0.20 mm mesh.

ii) Transfer 100 mg sample to 100 ml conical flasks to which 50 ml of bromocresole purple working solution (at the concentration of 0.13 mg/ml and acidity of 0.03 mol HCl/ml) is added.

iii) Stir the mixtures using a magnetic stirrer for 30 minutes.

iv) The content of the flask is centrifuge for 10 minutes (at 3000 rad/minutes).

v) Transfer 1 ml of clear extract to the tube containing 20 ml of 0.02 mol NaOH, mix and after 10 minutes measure the absorbance of the solution at 590 nm against distilled water as a reference.

Calculation

The mass of adsorbed active substance-bromocresole purple (equal to the value of the so-called bromocresole purple index-BCPI for each sample) is calculated as a difference between its quantity in the solution before and after contact with the ground sample. Determination is carried out by the measurement of absorbance of bromocresole purple colour solution using the proportional relationship between its concentration and absorbance at the wavelength of 590 nm.

The quantity of dye adsorbed – S (mg/g), which equals the value of BCPI for each sample, is calculated using equation following equation, and expressed per protein mass unit in dry matter of sample.

$$S = (Eo - Eb) \times C \times V / (Eo \times m)$$

Where: Eo is the absorbance of working solution, Eb is the absorbance of extract, C is the concentration of dye solution (0.13 mg/ ml), V is the volume of dye solution (50 ml) and m is the weight of sample (g).

16.2. Tannin determination

A. Vanillin assay

The vanillin assay is widely employed as a method for the quantitative determination of condensed tannins in fruits, sorghum and forage legumes (Broadhurst and Jones, 1978; Price *et al.*, 1978a). The principle of the assay is based on the substitution of vanillin for a phenolic hydroxyl group, yielding a red coloured condensation product which is measured spectrophotometrically at 480 to 550 nm.

a) Reagents

i) 1% vanillin in methanol (1.0 g vanillin up to 100 ml with absolute methanol). Store in a dark bottle at 4 °C.

ii) 8% concentrated HCl in methanol (8.0 ml concentrated HCl brought to 100 ml with absolute methanol).

iii) 4% concentrated HCl in methanol (4.0 ml concentrated HCl brought to 100 ml with absolute methanol).

iv) 0.3 mg/ml catechin (3.0 mg catechin brought to 10.0 ml with absolute methanol). Store in a dark bottle at 4 °C for up to three days.

b) Preparation of working reagents

The working vanillin reagent must be prepared daily from the solutions described above. One part of the 1% vanillin solution is mixed with one part of the 8% HCl solution. The working vanillin reagent and the 4% HCl solution are brought to 30 °C in the water bath before starting the analysis.

c) Extraction

For better results, the extraction and analysis should be carried out on a single day. The sample should be ground no more than one day in advance of analysis. About 200 g ground sample is weighed and extracted with 10.0 ml absolute methanol for 20 minutes in rotating scew cap culture tubes. The mixture is centrifuged for 10 minutes at 3000 g, and the supernatant is used in the analysis.

d) Analysis of standards

i) 0 to 1 ml aliquots of the catechin standard are dispensed into two sets of culture tubes and each sample is brought to 1 ml by the addition of absolute methanol. Tubes are incubated in the water bath.

ii) 5 ml of the working vanillin reagent is added at 1 minute intervals to one set of standards, and 5 ml of the 4% HCl solution is added at 1 minute intervals to the second set of standards.

iii) The samples are left in the water bath for exactly 20 minutes, and are then removed and the absorbance at 500 nm is read.

iv) Because the colour continues to develop as time passes, you cannot go back and re-read any sample. You must maintain the strict 1.0 minute intervals for reading that used in the addition of reagents.

The absorbance of the blank (vanillin reagent with no catechin) is subtracted from the absorbance of the corresponding vanillin containing sample. A standard curve is constructed and the linear portion of the curve is extrapolated to produce the standard curve.

e) Analysis of sample

i) 1 ml aliquots of each extract are dispensed into culture tubes. Duplicates of each sample are required so that the sample and a blank can be run for each sample.

ii) Tubes are incubated in the water bath at 30 °C.

iii) 5 ml of the vanillin reagent is added at 1 minute intervals to one set of samples and 5 ml of the 4% HCl solution is added at 1 minute intervals to the second set of the samples (the blank).

iv) The samples are left in the water bath for exactly 20 minutes and read at 500 nm absorbance.

Calculation

The absorbance of the blank is subtracted from the absorbance of the corresponding vanillin-containing sample. The value obtained is compared to the standard curve to obtain "catechin equivalents".

B. Folin-Denis assay

Tannin like compounds reduces phosphotungstomolybdic acid in alkaline solution to produce a highly coloured blue solution, the intensity of which is proportional to the amount of tannins. The intensity is measured in a spectrophotometer at 700 nm. The Folin-Denis assay is the most widely used type for measuring total phenol content in plant products. The principle is based on the reduction of phosphomolybdic- phosphotungstic acid (Folin-Denis reagent) to a blue colour complex in alkaline solution by phenols (Folin and Denis, 1912). This assay is relatively non-specific as it also reacts with several other compounds including xanthine, proteins and some amino acids. Tannic acid is commonly used as a standard. A second limitation of the Folin-Denis method is that it does not yield stoichiometric results, even when the number of hydroxyl groups is taken into account.

a) Reagents

i) Preparation of Folin-Denis reagent: Dissolve 100 g of sodium tungstate and 20 g of phosphomolybdic acid in 750 ml distilled water and later 50 ml phosphoric acid is added into the solution. Reflux mixture for 2 hrs and made volume to 1 l with distilled water.

ii) Preparation of carbonate solution: Dissolve 350 g of sodium carbonate in 1 l distilled water at 70 °C. Allow solution to stand overnight and then filtered it through glass-wool.

iii) Preparation of standard tannic acid solution: Dissolve 100 g of tannic acid in 100 ml distilled water.

iv) Preparation of working solution: Dilute 5 ml stock solution with 100 ml distilled water (each ml contains 50 μg of tannic acid).

b) Extraction of tannin

Weight 0.5 g of ground feed material and transfer to a 250 ml conical flask. Heat the flask gently and boil for 30 minutes. Centrifuged at 2,000 rpm for 20 minutes and collect the supernatant in 100 ml volumetric flask and make up the volume. Transfer 1 ml of the sample extract to a 100 ml volumetric flask containing 75 ml water. Add 5 ml of Folin-Denis reagent, 10 ml of sodium carbonate solution and dilute to 100 ml with water and shake well. Read the absorbance at 760 nm after 30 minutes incubation at room temperature.

c) Preparation of standard curve

10 ml of standard solution is made up to 100 ml with distilled water. Take 1 to 10 ml aliquots in clear test tubes and add 0.5 ml of Folin-Denis reagent and 1.0 ml of sodium carbonate solution to each tube. Make volume of each tube upto 10 ml with distilled water. All the reagents in each tube are mix well and kept undisturbed for about 30 minutes and read at 760 nm against reagent blank.

Calculation: The tannin concentration is determined by the standard graph of tannic acid solution.

C. Prussian blue assay

Prussian blue assay is used for total phenols estimation in representative samples. This assay is based on the reduction of the ferric ion (Fe^{3+}) to the ferrous ion (Fe^{2+}) by tannins and other phenolic compounds to form ferric ferrocyanide (Fe(III) [Fe(II) $(CN)_6]^-$), which is known as Prussian blue. The absorption of this complex can be measured at 720 nm (Price and Butler, 1977). Polyphenolics with a varying hydroxylation pattern and degree of polymerization react differently in this assay.

a) Reagents

i) 0.10 M $FeNH_4(SO_4)_2$ in 0.10 M HCl: Dilute concentrated HCl to 0.10 M by bringing 8.3 ml of the concentrated acid to 1 l with distilled water. Make the ferric ammonium sulfate by dissolving 48.2 g of the dodecahydrate salt (Fe $NH_4(SO_4)_2$. 12 H_2O in 1 l of the 0.10 M HCl. This will make a pale yellow solution.

ii) 0.008 M $K_3Fe(CN)_6$: Dissolve 2.63 g of potassium ferricyanide in 1 l of distilled water (this will make a yellow solution).

b) Determination

i) Dispense 0.10 ml sample (or a smaller appropriate volume of sample made up to 0.10 ml with sample solvent) into a 125 ml Erlenmeyer flask.

ii) Add 50.0 ml distilled (deionized) water. Poor quality water, especially iron-containing water, will give high blanks and unacceptable results.

iii) Add 3.0 ml Fe NH_4 $(SO_4)_2$ and swirl. Additions should be timed; 1 minute intervals are convenient.

iv) Exactly 20 minutes after the addition of the ferric ammonium sulfate, start timed (1 minute intervals) additions of 3.0 ml K_3Fe $(CN)_6$ swirl.

v) Exactly 20 minutes after the addition of the ferricyanide, read absorbance at 720 nm, making readings at 1 minute intervals.

vi) Include solvent-only blanks.

vii) Subtract the absorbance of the blank from the absorbance obtained for each sample. Standardize against 0.01 M gallic acid (0.094 g gallic acid monohydrate per 50 ml methanol).

D. Acid butanol assay

The acid butanol assay is a functional group assay which is specific for proanthocyanidins (condensed tannins), when used under the conditions described by Porter *et al.* (1986). The original procedure was described by Bate-Smith (1973). In this assay flavonoid subunits of the condensed tannins are oxidatively cleaved to yield anthocyanidin, which is measured spectrophotometrically. The method measures the total amount of subunits in the condensed tannin fraction.

a) Reagents

i) Acid butanol: Mix 950 ml of *n*-butanol with 50 ml concentrated HCl.

ii) Iron reagent: 2% Ferric ammonium sulfate in 2 N HCl. Bring 16.6 ml of concentrated HCl up to 100 ml with distilled water to make 2 N HCl. Dissolve 0.5 g $FeNH_4(SO_4)_2$. 12 H_2O in 25 ml of 2 N HCl. Store in a dark bottle.

b) Determination

i) In a 13 x 100 mm screw cap culture tube add 6.0 ml of the acid butanol reagent to a 1.0 ml aliquot of the sample (or a smaller volume of the sample made up to 1.0 ml with the sample solvent).

ii) Add 0.2 ml of the iron reagent, and vortex the sample. Cap the tube loosely, and put in a boiling water bath for 50 minutes.

iii) Cool the tube and read the absorbance at 550 nm. Subtract the absorbance of a blank containing only sample solvent, acid butanol and iron from the sample absorbance.

iv) Because water decreases the colour yield in this reaction, the reaction must be standardized with standard dissolved in exactly the solvent that the samples are to be dissolved in. Non aqueous samples will give the greatest colour, but the assay is sensitive enough to give adequate results even with substantial amounts of water present.

v) Standardize the assay with an appropriate proanthocyanidin, for example 1 mg/ml Sorghum tannin.

None of the colorimetric assays for tannin determination is very specific. Most of them, however, are appropriate for screening purposes, with the vanillin and acid butanol assays being most widely used.

E. Radial diffusion assay

The radial diffusion method (Hagerman, 1987) is a simple protein precipitation method and unlike other protein precipitation methods, acetone does not inhibit the precipitation reaction so acetone containing extracts can be conveniently assayed with this method.

a) Materials

i) Buffer: 0.05 M acetate containing 60 μM ascorbic acid; pH 5.0. For 1 l, dilute 2.85 ml glacial acetic acid to about 800 ml, add 10.6 mg ascorbic acid, and adjust pH to 5.0 with 2N NaOH. Then bring final volume to 1 l with water.

ii) Agarose: Type I, low EEO, gel point 36 °C.

iii) Bovine Serum Albumin (BSA): Fraction V powder, 96 to 99 % albumin.

iv) Disposable petri dishes (nominally 10 cm, actual diameter about 8.5 cm). Can be washed and reused numerous times.

v) 4.0 mm well punch.

vi) Parafilm

vii) Water bath, hot plate/stirrer, refrigerator, 30 °C incubator.

b) Preparation of plates

i) To make 8 to 9 plates (32 to 36 samples), add 1.0 g agarose to 100 ml of buffer in a 150 ml glass beaker.

ii) Heat with continuous stirring until the agarose dissolves. The solution will boil, and must not be allowed to boil over.

iii) Put the hot solution into the water bath set at 45 °C. Allow the agarose solution to cool, with occasionally stirring, to 45 °C. If the solution is not adequately cooled, the BSA will denature when it is added. If the solution is cooled too much, the agarose will set and the mixture must be re melted. After the BSA has been added the mixture cannot be re melted because the protein will be denatured.

iv) When the solution has reached 45 °C, add 0.10 g BSA with stirring. The BSA should be completely dissolved without allowing the solution to cool.

v) Using a 10.0 ml serological pipette with a large tip opening, dispense 9.5 ml of solution per plate. Dispense the solution carefully into the petri dishes. Do not allow the solution to bubble, and be sure that the surface of each dish is covered by solution. Allow the solution to harden while the dishes are on a level surface.

vi) Cover each dish and seal with a strip of parafilm. Store at 4 °C for up to several days before use. The layer of agarose in the dish should be of uniform thickness and free of bubbles or other imperfections.

c) Assay

i) Punch wells in each plate. Arrange the wells so there are four per plate, as far apart as possible. Use only gentle suction to remove the plugs of agarose, since you want uniform wells.

ii) Using a 10 µl glass syringe or a micropipette, apply the sample in 8 µl aliquots to the wells.

iii) The sample can be dissolved in any solvent that is convenient. Aqueous solutions evaporate and penetrate the wells very slowly and are less convenient than aqueous organic mixtures. The surface tension of pure organic solvents is low making it difficult to dispense the solutions. 50% methanol to be easiest to handle, but also frequently use 70% acetone.

iv) If the tannin is very dilute, 8 µl may not be sufficient for a response. You can add larger volumes by dispensing repetitive 8 µl samples. You must not allow the well to become completely dry between successive aliquots that are to be added.

v) After applying the samples, cover the plates and again seal with parafilm. Place the plates in a level incubator at 30 °C. Allow the rings to form for at least 96 hrs. Remove the plates, uncover, and use a plastic ruler to estimate the diameter of the ring that has formed. The square of the diameter is proportional to the amount of tannin in the sample.

vi) The plates can be stored after development at 4 °C for several weeks after sealing with parafilm.

16.3. Methods for nitrates and nitrites analysis

A. Quick field nitrate testing

A quick field test of forage nitrate concentration can be a useful tool to quickly screen whether additional laboratory testing for nitrates is warranted.

i) Presence of nitrate can be tested by using solution containing 0.5 g of diphenylamine in 20 ml of distilled water with 80 ml of concentrated sulphuric acid. Keep this solution in amber dropper bottles to protect the solution from light.

ii) Split stems of green fodder and other coarse grasses and drop the solution on the exposed stalk near the base. Nitrate tends to accumulate there, so low levels in the lower stem generally indicate low levels throughout the shoot.

Confirmation: Development of a blue colour indicates the presence of at least 10,000 ppm (1%) nitrate concentrations in the stalk. If a dark blue colour develops within a few seconds, whole plant samples should be collected and further analyzed for more precise testing of nitrate content by using laboratory method.

B. Laboratory testing for nitrates

Nitrate is reduced to nitrite by zinc and manganese sulphate. The reaction then consists of diazotisation of sulfonic acid by the nitrite ion and subsequent coupling with 1-naphthylamine to form a red dye. Copper aids the reaction at low ppm level (0.2) but over 1.2 ppm it interferes. Interfering iron is complexed with citrate. Reaction is optimum at pH range 1.7 to 3.0.

a) Reagents

i) 20% acetic acid reagent: 200 ml acetic acid, 5 ml copper sulphate (0.1572 g $CuSO_{4.}$ $5H_2O$, w/v) and diluted it to 1 l with distilled water.

ii) Brays indicator: a) 100 g barium sulphate ($BaSO_4$), b) 10 g manganese sulphate ($MnSO_4$. H_2O), c) 2 g zinc (metallic zinc), d) 75 g citric acid, e) 4 g sulfanilic acid and f) 2 g 1-naphthylamine. Zinc and citric acid are powdered, manganese sulphate, zinc, sulfanilic acid and 1-naphthylamine are mixed separately with a part of barium sulphate and then mixed with citric acid and remaining part of barium sulphate. The indicator is stored in blackened bottle away from light.

iii) N/10 hydrochloric acid.

iv) Activated charcoal.

v) Standard nitrate solution: stock solution: 1.37 g sodium nitrate in 1 l distilled water (nitrate = 1 mg/ml).

vi) Working solution: Dilute 1 ml of stock solution to 100 ml with distilled water (10 µg/ml).

b) Analysis

i) Moist sample (silage) kept frozen until analyzed. Dry green samples immediately in an oven at 60 °C.

ii) Take 1 g air dried material or 3 to 5 g moist sample in a conical flask (150 ml capacity).

iii) Add 100 ml of N/10 HCl and shake the content occasionally for 1 hr.

iv) If the extract is strongly coloured it is to be decolorized with activated charcoal.

v) Filter the content through Whatman filter paper 1.

c) Procedure

Addition of reagents/chemical sample, blank or standard.

Addition of reagents/chemical sample, blank or standard

Reagents/chemicals	Sample	Blank	Standard (μg/ml)			
			10	7.5	5.0	2.5
Extract (ml)	1	0	0	0	0	0
Distilled water (ml)	0	1	0	0.25	0.5	0.75
Working standard (ml)	0	0	1	0.75	0.5	0.25
Reagent 1 (ml)	9	9	9	9	9	9
Brays indicator (g)	0.5	0.5	0.5	0.5	0.5	0.5

Shake well and keep away from strong light. Centrifuge at 3000 rpm for 5 minutes. Remove any film on top and take the clear red supernatant. Read absorbance at 520 nm wave length.

Calculation

$$\text{Total nitrate}(\mu g/ml) = \frac{\text{Conc. of total nitrate in final soln.}(\mu g/ml)\text{ from std curve}}{\text{g sample taken (DM basis)} \times 10}$$

$$\text{nitrite conc.}(\mu g/ml) = \frac{\text{Conc. of in final soln. as obtained from std curve}}{\text{g sample taken (DM basis)} \times 10}$$

Total nitrate includes nitrates and nitrites, both.

16.4. Determination of hydrocyanic acid

Test is delicate and rapidity of change in colour depends upon amount of free hydrocyanic acid (HCN) present (Hogg and Ahlgren, 1942). This test work well with fresh plant materials but relatively less sensitive to dry substance, particularly ground cereal grains and protein meals.

a) Reagents

i) Alkaline picrate solution: dissolve 25 g Na_2CO_3 and 5 g of picric acid in 1000 ml of distilled water.

ii) Chloroform.

iii) Colour standards: dissolve 0.241 g KCN in 100 ml of water. This gives a stock solution containing 0.1 mg HCN per ml.

b) Preparation of test paper

The test paper is prepared by cutting sheets of filter paper into strips of 10 to 12 cm long and 0.5 cm wide and saturates them with alkaline picrate solution. The test paper should be moist with alkaline picrate solution when used.

c) Sample preparation

The sample for the analysis of HCN is taken from that portion of the plant which is immediately below the uppermost leaf collar. As test material, actively growing, vigorous tillers of 5 to 7 inches in length can be used regardless of the height of growth of the remaining portion of the plant. The plant sample is to be chopped into pieces of 0.5 to 1.0 cm in length with scissors or macerated. The plant material is dried at 70 °C for converting HCN-p (hydrocyanic acid potential) from a fresh to a dry weight basis.

d) Procedure

i) Standard solution: prepare standard by taking 5 ml of the alkaline picrate solution and 5 ml of the KCN solution in a test tube. Heat for 5 minutes in boiling water. Add 0, 0.1, 0.2, 0.4, 0.6, 0.8, 1.0 and 1.6 ml of KCN alkaline picrate solution to 8 test tubes, respectively. Bring the volume of each test tube up to 10 ml by adding distilled water. Stopper the tube and keep them in a cool and dark place.

ii) Place approximately 0.15 g of processed plant material in a test tube and add 3 to 4 drops of chloroform.

iii) Suspend a strip of moist filter paper saturated with sodium picrate solution above the mixture content of test tube.

iv) The test tube with content and filter paper strip is incubated at 20 °C temperature for 12 to 24 hrs.

v) The sodium picrate present in the filter paper is reduced to a reddish compound in proportion to the amount of HCN disolved.

vi) The colour produced is dissolved by placing the paper in a clean test tube containing 10 ml of distilled water after which the colour of the water is matched with colour standard at 510 nm wavelength.

vii) Similar to above, also run samples for blank (without test feed) and standards.

Calculation

$$\text{Total cyanide content (mg / kg)} = 396 \times \text{absorbance reading}$$

16.5. Determination of total oxalate contents

A. Spectrophotometric method

a) Oxalate extraction

i) Homogenize 1.5 g of sample with 1.6 ml 0.5 mol/l HCl first, and then dilute with 1 ml distilled water.

ii) Transfer homogenate into 10 ml graduated tubes and heat in a boiling water bath for 20 minutes.

iii) After cooling, add distilled water to each tube to bring the volume of homogenate upto 10 ml.

iv) Incubate for overnight at room temperature.

v) The next day, clarify 1 ml of homogenate by centrifugation at 12, 000 g for 10 minutes at 4 °C.

vi) After this, add 0.016 ml NaOH (2 mol/l) to 0.5 ml supernatant (this mixture is termed as oxalate extract).

b) Oxalate determination

i) Add 20 mg of oxalate oxidase in the form of dry powder (prepared from wheat bran) in a 2 ml test tube.

ii) Add 0.1 ml distilled water; 0.8 ml colour reagent (contains 10 mg of 4-aminoantipyrine, 25 μl of N, N-dimethylaniline per 100 ml of 125 mmol/l succinate-NaOH buffer with 75% alcohol (v/v), pH 4.0) and 0.04 ml (150 U/ml) horseradish peroxidase are added before 0.1 ml oxalate extract is added to initiate the reaction.

iii) Take absorbance of the reaction mixture at 555 nm in a spectrophotometer after incubation at room temperature for 90 minutes.

iv) Determine oxalate content with reference to the standard curve which is prepared by adding 0, 2, 4, 6, 8, and 10 μg oxalic acid into 1 ml reaction system, respectively. The unit of oxalate is presented as mean mg oxalate/100 g fresh weight feed material.

B. Chromatography method

a) Sample preparation

i) Dry representative feed and faecal samples in a oven at 65 °C for a minimum of 48 hrs.

ii) Grind dried samples using a Wiley, mill to pass through a 0.5 mm screen.

iii) Place 0.2 g sample in a 16 mm glass test tube fitted with a plastic cap and add 5 ml of extraction methylation solution (comprised 100 ml of a 2:1 mixture of anhydrous chloroform and absolute methanol to which 5 ml of concentrated sulphuric acid were added).

iv) Vortex sample, capped, then incubate overnight at room temperature.

v) Add 1 ml of distilled water and vortex the mixture.

vi) Filter content through phase separating filter paper.

vii) Use 0.2 μl aliquot of the organic filtrate for injection into gas chromatography for oxalate quantitation.

viii) Freeze dry 2 ml of acidified urine samples for 48 hrs. The pellet remaining after drying is process for oxalate determination in the same way as feed and faecal samples.

b) Oxalate quantitation

The total oxalate content in feed, faeces and acidified, freeze-dried urine is analyzing by method of Roughan and Slack (1973). The GC fitted with a 30 mm column (preferably Durabond Wax column) can be use for analysis. Keep oven temperature at 100 °C, kept injector ports and detectors 200 °C. Maintain nitrogen carrier gas at a pressure of 138 kPa. The split ratio should be 1:63.4. Determine peak areas on an integrator. Increase oven temperature to 175 °C after every 10 sample runs to eliminate residue accumulation in the column.

16.6. Determination of saponin

A. Qualitative tests

a) Saponin test with dry sample (Edeoga *et al.*, 2005): Dry feedstuffs for overnight at 60 °C and grind to powder by blender. Shake 0.5 g of crude powder with water in a test tube. Develop stable persistent froth while warming content in water bath. Add 3 drops of olive oil in frothy content and shake vigorously. Formation of emulsion indicates the presence of saponins.

b) Saponin test with fresh Sample (Edeoga *et al.*, 2005): Dissolve and blend 10 g of fresh sample in 100 ml distilled water (1:10) in a test tube. Filter the content and warm in water bath. Develop stable persistent froth while warming content in water bath. Add 3 drops of olive oil in frothy content and shake vigorously. Formation of emulsion indicates the presence of saponins.

B. Quantitative tests

i) Dry samples of feedstuffs for overnight at 60 °C and grind to a fine powder by blender.

ii) Take 1 g of dried sample and dissolve it in 20 ml of 20% isopropanol.

iii) Heat mixture at 86 °C during 20 minutes for saponin extraction using water bath and filter (using Whatman paper) for further quantification.

iv) Mix 1 ml of filtered sample solution with 3.5 ml Liebermann-Burchards (LB; consist of a 1:5 mixture of acetic acid and sulfuric acid, respectively) reagent. LB reagent is use for saponin quantification as it is capable of producing a light brown staining if these compounds are present in a sample.

v) Take absorbance of all samples at 580 nm after 10 minutes of incubation at room temperature.

Calculation

A calibration curve based on pure quinoa saponins is used to determine the final concentration of saponins (mg/ml) in each solution on the basis of absorbance measurements (Absorbance = 4.5725 × Concentration of saponins + 0.0164). The % saponin content is calculated on the basis of fresh weight.

16.7. Gossypol determination (Method; ISO 6866:1985)

Extraction of the gossypol in the presence of 3-aminopropan-1-01, either with a mixture of 2-propanol and hexane for the determination of free gossypol or with dimethylformamide for the determination of total gossypol. Conversion of the gossypol into gossypol-dianiline using aniline. Measurement of the absorbance at the wavelength of maximum absorbance (between 435 and 445 nm).

a) Reagents

i) 2-Propanol/*n*-hexane, 60 + 40 mixture by volume

ii) Solvent A: Place In a 1000 ml volumetric flask approximately 500 ml of the 2-propanol/hexane mixture, 2 ml of 3-aminopropan-1-ol, 8 ml of glacial acetic acid and 50 ml of water. Make up to volume with the 2-propanol/hexane mixture. This reagent is stable for one week only.

iii) Solvent B: Place in a 100 ml volumetric flask 2 ml of 3-aminopropan-1-ol and 10 ml of glacial acetic acid. Cool to room temperature and make up to volume with N, N-dimethylformamide. This reagent is stable for one week only.

iv) Aniline: If the absorbance determined in the blank test exceeds 0.022, distil the aniline over zinc dust, discarding the first and last 10% fractions of distillate. Store in a stoppered brown glass bottle in a refrigerator (0 to 4 °C). The reagent is stable for several months.

b) Procedure

The weight of the test sample depends on the expected gossypol content. For the determination of free gossypol in cottonseed and cottonseed meals and cakes the weight of the sample should not exceed 1 g for compound feeding stuffs, it may be as much as 5 g. For the determination of total gossypol, the weight of the test sample should be between 0.5 to 5 g.

i) Transfer the 1 to 5 g of test sample to a 250 ml conical flask, the bottom of which has been covered with glass beads.

ii) Add, by means of a pipette, 50 ml of solvent A. Stopper the flask and mix, using the tumbler mixer for 1 hr. Filter through a dry filter paper, collecting the filtrate in a 100 ml conical flask. During filtration, cover the funnel with a watch glass.

iii) Transfer, by means of a pipette, identical aliquot portions of the filtrate, containing 50 to 100 μg of gossypol, to each of two 25 ml volumetric flasks (C and D). If necessary, make up to 10 ml with solvent A.

iv) Make up the contents of flask C to volume with the 2-propanol/ hexane mixture and mix. This solution will be used as the reference solution against which the test solution will be measured.

v) Transfer, by means of a pipette, 10 ml of solvent A into each of two 25 ml volumetric flasks (E and F),

vi) Make up the contents of flask E to volume with the 2 propano/ hexane mixture and mix. This solution will be used as the reference solution against which the blank lest solution will be measured.

vii) Add 2 ml of the aniline to flasks D and F. Heat for 30 minutes on a boiling water-bath to develop the colour.

viii) Cool to room temperature, make up to volume with the 2-propanol/hexane mixture, mix and leave for 1 hr.

ix) Measure the absorbance of the blank test solution against the reference solution (flask F) and the absorbance of the test solution (flask D) against the reference solution (flask C) using the spectrometer at the wavelength of maximum absorbance (between 435 and 445 nm). Subtract the absorbance of the blank test solution from that of the test solution to obtain the corrected absorbance.

Determination of total gossypol

i) Transfer 5 g of test sample into a 50 ml volumetric flask and add 10 ml of solvent B.

ii) Transfer 10 ml of solvent B to a second 50 ml volumetric flask and heat the two flasks for 30 minutes on a boiling water-bath.

iii) Cool to room temperature and make up to volume with the 2-propanol/hexane mixture. Mix and leave to settle for 10 to 15 minutes, then filter and collect the filtrates in 50 ml conical flasks.

iv) Transfer, by means of a pipette, 2 ml of the filtrate obtained from the test portion, containing 40 to 200 µg of gossypol, into each of two 25 ml volumetric flasks and 2 ml of the filtrate obtained from the second flask into each of two other 25 ml volumetric flasks.

v) Make up the contents of one of the flasks containing the test solution and of one flask from the blank test to volume with the 2-propanol/hexane mixture.

vi) These solutions will be used as reference solutions,

vii) Add 2 ml of the aniline to the remaining test and blank test solutions. Heat for 30 minutes on a boiling water-bath to develop the colour. Cool to room temperature, make up to volume with the 2-propanol/hexane mixture, mix and leave for 1 hr.

viii) Measure the absorbance of the solutions at wavelength ranges between 435 to 445 nm.

Calculation

The free or total gossypol content, expressed in milligrams per kilogram of the product as received, is equal to

$$(A \times 1250 \times 1000) / (a \times m \times V) = (A \times 125) / (amV) \times 10^6$$

Where, A is the corrected absorbance, m is the mass in grams, of the test portion, V is the volume (ml) of the aliquot portion of filtrate taken and a is the specific mass absorbance coefficient (62.5 $cm^{-1} \times g^{-1}$ in case of free gossypol and 60 $cm^{-1} \times g^{-1}$ in case of total gossypol).

16.8. Determination of mycotoxin

A. Thin layer chromatography method

This method is applicable for determination of aflatoxins in ground maize, wheat, barley and other feed samples that does not have colouring substances other than carotenoids. It is suggested to grind 100 g of sample after drying (50 °C). Extract aflatoxins from 50 g of processed sample by using methanol: deionized water (80:20 v/v). For this, mix 50 g of sample with methanol: deionized water (80:20 v/v) for 30 minutes at 120 rpm using a shaker. Filter solution through filter paper and 20 ml of filtered solution is dilute 4:1 with phosphate buffer solution (pH, 7.4). The extract collected is further purified using column chromatography. Isolate the extract of aflatoxin by column chromatography. For this, apply 50 ml of the extract onto the column and allow to flow at a rate of 1 ml/minute. After the aflatoxin molecules were bound, wash column with diagnosed water in order to remove unbound materials. Then, elute aflatoxins by using 2 ml methanol. Incubate elute at 50 °C and evaporated by using nitrogen. The purified extract is condensed by evaporating and subjected to thin layer chromatography (TLC) for its determination. In the case of TLC the amount of aflatoxin B_1 is estimated visually by comparing fluorescence intensity of aflatoxin in the sample with that of known quantity of aflatoxin B_1 standard or more accurately by separating the fluorescent area from TLC plate and dissolving in methanol and comparing the intensity of aflatoxin B_1 at the spectrophotometer with different concentrations of standard.

a) Sample preparation

Aflatoxins are likely to occur in few pockets at high concentration which may not be randomly distributed. Perform sampling and sample preparation, keeping this point in mind. Due to possibility of pockets of contamination, include total laboratory sample (2 kg) in sample preparation. Aim at maximal particle size reduction and thoroughness of mixing to achieve effective distribution of contaminated portions.

b) Preparation of TLC plates

Plates are coated with silica gel slurry to a thickness of 0.25 to 0.30 mm using standard applicator. Air dry coated plates are activated for 2 hrs at 105 °C and store in a desiccating chamber until use.

i) Clean up column-300 mm × 10 mm long with 35 μm porous polyethylene frit with stopcock.

ii) Separating funnel (500 ml), beakers (500 ml and 100 ml), measuring cylinders, funnels, etc.

iii) Viewing chamber fitted with UV lamp having 360 nm wave lengths.

c) Reagents

i) Acetone, acetonitrile, benzene, chloroform, diethyl ether, *n*-hexane/petroleum ether (60 to 80 °C) and methanol.

ii) Column washes solvent-anhydrous, diethyl ether: *n*-hexane (3:1).

iii) Aflatoxin eluting solvent-chloroform: methanol (97:3).

iv) Standard aflatoxin dissolving solvent- benzene: acetonitrile (98:2).

v) Anhydrous sodium sulphate (Na_2SO_4).

vi) Silica gel for TLC (60 to 120 mesh): dry it in about 1 inch thick 10 layer for 2 hrs at 105 °C, cool in a vapour tight container at 1% water (1ml in 100g), shake well and equilibrate at least 15 hrs. Store in screw capped bottle in vapour tight container.

vii) Silica gel G for TLC (60 mesh).

viii) Aflatoxin standard solution: prepare a stock solution containing 20 µg/ml of B_1 from high purity crystalline B_1. From the stock solution prepare working standard containing 1 to 5 µg/ml aflatoxin B_1. Standard solution should be stored in well stoppered flask/tubes at 0 °C.

d) Protocol

i) 50 g finely ground feed sample is taken into an Erlenmeyer flask and mixed thoroughly with 25 ml distilled water with the help of glass rod to prevent lump formation. Add 250 ml of chloroform and shake on a wrist action shaker for 30 minutes. Filter the contents through Whatman filter paper 1 and collect 50 ml portion of clear filtrate. Condense the 50 ml portion on a water bath to 1 to 2 ml and save the concentrated portion for column clean up.

ii) Preparation of silica gel column: take a glass column of size 1 x 30 cm equipped with a sintered plate or place a ball of glass wool loosely in the bottom. Clamp it on a stand and add about 20 ml chloroform keeping the stopcock closed. Add in sequence from the bottom to top 1 g of anhydrous sodium sulphate, 2 g of silica gel (60 to 120 mesh) and 1.5 g of anhydrous sodium sulphate. When the three additives have formed proper layer, allow the solvent to run down. As soon as the chloroform crosses the top of the column load quantitatively the 2 ml concentrated extract of sample and allow it to percolate through the column. As soon as the sample crosses the top of the column bed, give washing to the material in the column with 75 ml of solvent mixture (diethyl ether: *n*-hexane, 3: 1) and discard it. When the washing is over, add 60 ml of the eluting solvent mixture prepared using the chloroform: methanol (97: 3). Collect this elute in a 100 ml conical flask.

iii) Evaporate until dry ether on rotary evaporator or on a water bath and transfer the residue quantitatively to a 5 ml vial. Make up the volume with benzene: acetonitrile or with chloroform to 0.2 ml. Shake well to dissolve the aflatoxin. Dissolved residue is now used for spotting on TLC plate.

iv) Prepare TLC plates using a slurry of silica gel G (60 mesh) in distilled water. A slurry prepared by mixing 12 g of silica gel G in 20 ml of distilled water is optimum to coat two plates of 20 x 20 cm size. Plate should be activated before spotting in an oven maintained at 105 ± 2 °C for 1 hr.

v) Spot 5 µl or less of the cleaned sample extract with suitable dilutions on to the silica gel plate along with 5 µl or less of aflatoxin B1 standard solution containing 2, 4 and 6 mg of toxin per 5 µl or less of solvent (Benzene: acetonitrile, 98: 2). Develop the plates in the following solvent systems (200 ml) independently.

a) Chloroform: acetone: methanol (90: 8: 2).

b) Chloroform: methanol (95: 5).

c) Toluene: isoamyl alcohol: methanol (66: 32: 2).

Allow the plates to develop for 30 to 40 minutes in anyone of the above solvent systems. Remove the plates, air dry and visualize the spots under long wave range UV cabinet, comparing the sample florescent spots with standard. After identifying the standard spot which just matches with the sample or the matched band of sample and standard is removed from plates and dissolve in 2 ml methanol and keep overnight. Centrifuge for 10 minutes. The supernatant is collected twice by adding 2 ml and 1 ml methanol. This final filtrate is used to note OD on the spectrophotometer at 363 nm along with standard using methanol as a blank.

Calculation

$$\text{Aflatoxin B1 content}(\mu g / kg) = \frac{A \times B \times C}{D \times E}$$

Where, A is the µl or OD of the aflatoxin B1 standard equal to that of sample material being evaluated on the plate, B is the concentration of aflatoxin B1 standard (µg/ml), C is the µl of solvent required to dilute final extract, D is the weight of dried sample in g, E is the µl of sample extract spotted to give fluorescence intensity equal to standard B1.

B. Immunoassay (Kawamura *et al.*, 1988)

Although most of chromatographic methods are sensitive and accurate, they are laborious, expensive, time consuming and unsuitable for analysis of large number of samples and also require costly equipment and extensive clean-up procedures. Fast, reliable and sensitive analytical methods are needed, due to the strict guidelines on mycotoxin contamination that have been imposed by importing countries. This demand has led to the development of quantitative or semi-quantitative methods for mycotoxin screening, based on immunochemical techniques, such as enzyme-linked immunosorbent assays (ELISAs), since they do not require costly instrumentation, are able to analyze a large number of samples simultaneously and require no sample clean-up. In general, ELISAs are rapid, simple, specific and sensitive; they can be used in the field and have become the most common rapid methods for mycotoxin detection in food and feed

a) Sample extraction

i) An aliquot of feed sample (2 g) is shaken for 10 minutes at 150 rpm with 10 ml methanol: water (70:30, v/v).

ii) The crude extract is then filtered through Whatman filter paper 1 and diluted in PBST (PBS + 0.05% Tween 20) for Intra-cellular (IC)-ELISA determination.

b) IC-ELISA determination

i) Coat 96 wells ELISA plate with 100 µl AFB_1-BSA (bovine serum albumin) in PBS (0.015 M, pH 7.3) at 4 °C for 18 hrs.

ii) Wash microtitre plates five times after each incubation step with PBST.

iii) In order to minimize non-specific binding, block wells with 200 μl 0.1% ovalbumin in PBS at 37 °C for 1 hr.

iv) After the washing step, add 50 μl anti-aflatoxin B_1 monoclonal antibody and 50 μl AFB_1 standards (0.05 to 10 ng/ml) or feed extracts and incubated at 25 °C for 1 hr.

v) Following a washing step, add 100 μl horseradish peroxidase labelled goat anti-mouse IgG and incubated at 25 °C for 1 hr.

vi) Wash again and add 100 μl substrate solutions (H_2O_2).

vii) After 20 minutes, stop the reaction by adding 50 μl 1M H_2SO_4.

Calculation

Measure the absorbance of each well at 450 nm in an ELISA microplate reader. The average absorbance is calculated from the individual absorbances obtained from triplicate wells and the results are expressed as percentage of binding:

$$\text{Binding}(\%) - \frac{\text{Ap}}{\text{An}} \times 100$$

Where, Ap is the mean absorbance in the presence of the aflatoxin standard or feed extract sample and An is the mean absorbance in their absence.

❑❑❑

17

Determination of Pesticide Residues

Any substance or mixture of substances intended for preventing, destroying, or controlling any pest, including vectors of human or animal disease, unwanted species of plants or animals, causing harm during or otherwise interfering with the production, processing, storage, transport, or marketing of food, agricultural commodities, wood and wood products or animal feedstuffs, or substances that may be administered to animals for the control of insects, arachnids, or other pests in or on their bodies. The term pesticide includes herbicide, insecticide, insect growth regulator, nematicide, termiticide, molluscicide, piscicide, avicide, rodenticide, predacide, bactericide, insect repellent, animal repellent, antimicrobial, fungicide, antimicrobial disinfectant, and sanitizer. The most common of these are herbicides which account for approximately 80% of all pesticide use.

Determination of organochlorine pesticide residues by gas chromatographic-method

a) Extraction (Bennett *et al.*, 1997)

i) Blend about 50 g sample with 350 ml acetonitrile: water mixture (65:35) for 5 minutes at high speed, (the addition of water to acetonitrile increases the extractability of organochlorine pesticide residues in dry fodders and straws) and filter with the help of filter paper (Whatman filter paper 1) into 500 ml conical flask.

ii) Transfer the filtrate to 250 ml graduated cylinder and record the volume.

iii) Transfer the filtrate into 1000 ml separating funnel.

iv) Measure 100 ml petroleum ether and pour into the separating funnel.

v) Shake vigorously (1 to 2 minutes) and add about 10 ml saturated sodium chloride solution and 600 ml of water mixed gently and thoroughly.

vi) Allow to separate.

vii) Discard aqueous layer and washed the solvent layer twice with 100 ml portions of water. Discard washings.

viii) Transfer the solvents to 100 ml stoppered graduated cylinder and recorded the volume.

ix) This solvent is concentrated to 5 to 10 ml before it is passed through the column.

x) Extract the concentrated mixture and feed ingredients for OCPRs along with fat by the Soxhlet extraction. About 0.5 g extracted fat was dissolved in 5 ml portion of petroleum ether and passed through a column containing florisil for separation.

xi) The extract is ready for column chromatography, on partially deactivated florisil cartridges.

b) GC analysis

The cleaned up residues were measured using a gas chromatograph equipped with ECD.

Column - Equity TM -5, 30 m x 0.25 mm ID x 0.25 μm

c) Operating conditions of GC

1.	Injection port temperature	225 °C
2.	Column oven temperature	100°C (2 minutes), 15 to 160°C/ minute, 5 to 300°C/minute (10 minutes)
3.	Detector temperature	310 °C
4.	Carrier gas	Helium, 30 cm/second @ 100 °C
5.	Total run time	35 minutes

Calculation

$$\text{Pesticide residues } (\mu g / l) - \frac{A \times B \times C \times D}{E \times F \times G}$$

Where, A is the ng of standard pesticide, B is the peak area of sample, C is the extracted volume (μl) D is the dilution factor, E is the peak area of standard, F is the volume of extract injected (μl) and G is the volume of sample extracted (ml).

□□□

REFERENCES

Association of Official Analytical Chemists. 1995. Official Methods of Analysis. 16th ed. AOAC. Washington DC.

Barker, S. B., Summerson, W.H. 1941. The colorimetric determination of lactic acid in biological material. Journal of biological Chemistry, 138: 535.

Bate-Smith, E.C. 1973. Tannins in herbaceous leguminosae. Phytochemistry, 12: 1809–1812.

Bennett, D.A., Chung, A.C., Lee S.M. 1997. Multi residue method for analysis of pesticides in liquid whole milk. Journal of Association of Official Analytical Chemical International, 80: 1065.

Broadhurst, R.B., Jones, W.T. 1978. Analysis of condensed tannins using acidified vanillin. Journal of the Science of Food and Agriculture, 29: 788-794.

Celio Pasquini. 2003. Near infrared spectroscopy: fundamentals, practical aspects and analytical applications. Journal of the Brazilian Chemical Society, 14(2): 198-219.

Chandrasekaran Natarajan, C.A., Sundram, T.K. 2001. Physical evaluation of feed ingredients in Hand book of poultry nutrition, American Soybean Association India.

Chawla, R., Kaur, H. 2001. Isocratic HPLC method for simultaneous determination of beta carotene, retinol and alfa tocopherol in feeds and blood plasma. Indian Journal of Dairy Science, 54: 84-90.

Edeoga H.O., Okwu, D.E., Mbaeble B.O. 2005. Phytochemical constituents of some Nigerian medicinal plants. African Journal of Biotechnology, 4: 685- 688.

Eirenmiller, R.R., Landen, W.O. 1998. In: Vitamin analysis for the health and food sciences. CRC Press Inc. Pp. 518.

Folin, O., Denis, W. 1915. Journal of Biological Chemistry, XXII, 309.

Garg, M.R., Sherasia, P.L., Bhanderi, B.M. 2013. Quality control manual for cattle feed plants. Animal Nutrition Group, National Dairy Development Board, Anand.

Hagerman, A.E. 1987. Radial diffusion method for determining tannin in plant extracts. Journal of Chemical Ecology, 13: 437.

Hogg, P.G., Ahlgren, H.L. 1942. A rapid method for determining hydrocyanic acid content of single plants of sudan grass. Journal of the American Society of Agronomy, 34: 199-200.

IS 15120: 2002. Animal feeding stuffs-determination of vitamin A content-method using high performance liquid chromatography.

ISO 14902: 2001(E). 2001. Animal feed Stuffs- determination of trypsin inhibitor activity of soya products.

ISO 6866-1985. 1986. Methods for analysis of animal feeding stuffs-determination of gossypol.

Johnson, K.A., Westberg, H.H., Michal, J.J., Cossalman, M.W. 2007. The SF_6 Tracer Technique: Methane measurement from ruminants. Pp. 33-67.

Joseph, J.D., Ackman, R.G. 1992. Capillary column gas chromatography method for analysis of encapsulated fish oil and fish oil ethyl esters: collaborative study. Journal of Association of Official Analytical Chemical International, 75: 488-506.

Jouany, J.P. 1981. Dosages des acides gras volatils et des alcools dans les ensilages par chromatographie en phase gazeuse. Bulletin *technique* du *CRZV* de Theix- INRA, 46: 63-66.

Kawamura, O., Nagayama, S., Sato, S., Ohtani, K., Ueno, I., Ueno, Y. 1988. A monoclonal antibody-based enzyme-linked immunosorbent assay of aflatoxin B_1 in peanut products. Mycotoxin Research, 4: 75–87.

Khajaren, J., Khajaren, S. 1998. Quick quality test for protein meals. Technical Bulletin, American Soybean Association.

Khajaren, J., Sinchermsiri D., Hanbunchong A. 1987. Manual feed microscopy and quality control. Dhornhvaj Co., Ltd. Bangkok, Thailand.

Makkar, H.P.S., Blummel, M., Borowy, N.K, Becker, K. 1993. Gravimetric determination of tannins and their correlations with chemical and protein precipitation methods. Journal of the Science of Food and Agriculture, 61: 161-165.

Menke, K.H., Raab, L., Salweski, A., Steingass, H., Fritz, D., Schneider, W. 1979. The estimation of the digestibility and metabolizable energy content of ruminant feedstuffs from the gas production when they are incubated with rumen liquor *in vitro*. The Journal of Agricultural Science, 93: 217-222.

Menke, K.H., Steingass, H. 1988. Estimation of the energetic feed values obtained from chemical analysis and in vitro gas production using rumen fluid. Animal Research and Development, 28: 7-55.

Nordlund, K.V., Garrett, E.F. 1994. Rumenocentesis: a technique for the diagnosis of subacute rumen acidosis in dairy herds. Bovine Practitioner, 28: 104.

Norris, K.H., Hart, J.R. 1965. Direct spectroscopic determination of moisture content of grain and seeds; humidity moisture, pp. 19. In: Principles and methods of measuring in liquids and solids, ed. By P.N. Winn, Jr., Reinhold Pub. Corp., New York.

Ørskov, E.R., McDonald, I. 1979. The estimation of protein degradability in the rumen from incubation measurements weighted according to rates of passage. The Journal of Agricultural Science, 92: 499–503.

Porter, L.J., Hirstich, L.N., Chan, B.G. 1986. The conversion of procyanidins and prodelphinidins to cyanidin and delphinidin. Phytochemistry, 25: 223–230.

Price, M.L., Butler, L.G., 1977. Rapid visual estimation and spectrophotometric determination of tannin content of sorghum grain. Journal of Agriculture and Food Chemistry, 25: 1268–1273.

Price, M.L., Van Scoyoc, S., Butler, L.G. 1978a. A critical evaluation of the vanillin reaction as an assay for tannin in sorghum grain. Journal of Agricultural and Food Chemistry, 26: 1214-1218.

Roughan, P.G., Slack, C.R. 1973. Simple methods for routine screening and quantitative estimation of oxalate content of tropical grasses. The Journal of the Science of Food and Agriculture, 24: 803-811.

Spelbrink, R.E.J., Gerrits, P.J., Mooj, C., Giuseppin, M.L.F. 2011. Quantitative determination of trypsin inhibitory activity in complex matrices. The Open Food Science Journal, 5: 42-46.

Sukhija, P.S., Palmquist, D.L. 1988. Rapid method for determination of total fatty acid content and composition of feedstuffs and feces. Journal of Agricultural and Food Chemistry, 36: 1202–1206.

Szmigielski, M., Matyka, S. 2004. Comparison of selected methods appled for the evaluation of thermal processing efficiency of chickling vetch seeds. Polish Journal of Food and Nutrition Sciences, 13/54 (3): 243-248.

Talapatra, S.K., Ray, S.C., Sen, K.C. 1940. Estimation of phosphorous, chloride, calcium, sodium and potassium in food stuffs. Indian Journal of Veterinary Science, 10: 243–258.

Taylor, K.A.C.C. 1996. A simple colorimetric assay for muramic acid and lactic acid. Applied Biochemistry and Biotechnology, 56(1): 49-58.

USAID. 2016. Predict Operating Procedures: Livestock Sampling. Pp. 17.

Van Soest, P.J. 1963. Use of detergents in the analysis of fibrous feeds. I. Preparation of fibre residues of low nitrogen content. Journal of the Association of Official Agricultural Chemists, 46: 825–829.

Weatherburn, M.W. 1967. Phenol-hypochlorite reaction for determination of ammonia. The Journal of Analytical Chemistry, 39: 971–974.

❑❑❑

Appendices

APPENDIX I

LIST OF ABBREVIATIONS

%	Percentage	IU	International unit
°C	Degree celsius	IVGPT	*In vitro* gas production technique
μg	Micro gram	kg	Kilo gram
μl	Micro litre	l	Litre
AAS	Atomic absorption spectrophotometry	L-BAPA	Benzoyl-L-arginine-p-nitroanilide
ADF	Acid detergent fibre	M	Molarity
ADFCP	Acid detergent fibre crude protein	m	Molality
ADIN	Acid detergent insoluble nitrogen	MBP	Microbial biomass production
ADL	Acid detergent lignin	Mcal	Mega calorie
ADS	Acid detergents solution	ME	Metabolizable energy
AIA	Acid insoluble ash	mg	Milligram
ANFs	Anti-nutritional factors	mm	Millimeter
AOAC	Association of Official Analytical Chemists	mol	Mole
BCAA	Branched chain amino acids	Mol. wt.	Molecular weight

BCPI	Bromocresol purple index	N	Normality
BIS	Bureau of Indian Standard	NDF	Neutral detergent fibre
BSA	Bovine serum albumin	NDS	Neutral detergent solution
cc	Cubic centimeters	NFE	Nitrogen free extract
CF	Crude fibre	ng	Nano gram
CH_4	Methane	NH_3-N	Ammonia nitrogen
CP	Crude protein	NIR	Near-infrared
DC	Digestibility coefficient	NPN	Non protein nitrogen
DE	Digestible energy	OM	Organic matter
DM	Dry matter	pg	Pico gram
EE	Ether extract	ppb	Parts per billion
ECD	Electron capture detector	ppm	Parts per million
ELISA	Enzyme-linked immunosorbent assays	RUSITEC	Rumen simulation technique
Eq. wt.	Equivalent weight	SAA	Sulphur amino acids
FAAS	Flame atomic absorption spectrophotometry	SF_6	Sulphur hexafluoride
FAMEs	Fatty acid methyl esters	TCA	Trichloroacetic acid
g	Gram	TDDM	True degradability of dry matter
G	Gauge	TDN	Total digestible nutrients
GC	Gas chromatography	TDOM	True degradability of organic matter
GE	Gross energy	TIA	Trypsin inhibitor activity
GFAAS	Graphite furnace atomic absorption spectrometry	TLC	Thin layer chromatography
GHG	Green house gas	TMR	Total mixed ration
GLC	Gas liquid chromatography	v/v	Volume/volume

HPLC	High performance liquid chromatography	VFA	Volatile fatty acid
hr(s)	Hour(s)	w/v	Weight/volume
ICP-AES	Inductively coupled plasma-atomic emission spectrometry	w/w	Weight/weight
ISO	International Standard Organization		

APPENDIX II

NUTRIENT COMPOSITION OF COMMON FEEDSTUFFS

Ingredient	ME (Kcal/ kg)	Crude protein (%)	Crude fiber (%)	Ether extract (%)	Lysine (%)	Methio-nine (%)	Calcium (%)	Phosp-horus (%)
Cereals								
Maize	3309	9.2	3.0	3.8	0.18	0.15	0.25	0.40
Bajra	2950	12.7	4.0	3.0	0.43	0.20	0.13	0.72
Wheat	3045	10.3	3.0	2.5	0.47	0.21	0.19	1.12
Rice	2345	7.9	8.0	2.5	0.33	0.17	0.11	0.48
Barely	2618	12.0			0.60	0.20	0.29	0.64
Cereal by product								
Rice polish	2837	12.7	12.0	16.0	0.55	0.24	0.27	1.37
De-oiled rice polish	2135	14.1	14.0	1.0	0.44	0.31	0.37	1.80
Wheat bran	1286	17.2	10.9	3.0	0.53	0.09	0.19	1.12
Vegetable protein								
Soybean meal	2300	45.0	6.0	1.0	2.57	0.76	0.36	0.90
Full fat soybean	3275	36.5	5.5	18.0	2.35	0.53	0.25	0.58
Groundnut cake	2700	38.0	9.0	8.0	1.6	0.42	0.16	0.16
Groundnut ext.	2128	40-42	11.2	1.0	1.47	0.68	0.31	0.67
Sunflower cake	1600	28.0	26.0	1.0	1.00	0.60	0.37	0.30

Mustard cake	2373	35.1	9.6	8.0	1.14	0.42	0.89	1.78
De-oiled mustard cake	1672	31.7	11.6	2.3	1.37	0.51	0.58	0.82
Cotton seed meal	1556	25.9	21.3	0.9	1.07	0.41	0.52	0.86
Guar meal	1821	37.1	10.5	6.7	2.58	0.39	0.41	0.50
Maize gluten meal	3300	60.0	2.0	2.5	1.02	1.28	0.22	0.19
Brewer's dried grains	2732	28.2	-	-	0.98	0.43	0.29	0.54
Animal proteins								
Fish meal	1834	43.1	2.5	6.0	2.5	1.08	7.16	2.5
Meat meal	2300	56.2	2.6	6.8	4.00	0.84	2.68	2.06
Meat cum bone meal	2100	48.0	-	8.0	3.72	0.75	11.25	5.39
Mineral source								
DCP	-	-	-	-	-	-	23	18
Limestone	-	-	-	-	-	-	35.0	-
Oyster shell	-	-	-	-	-	-	38.0	-

UNITS AND CONVERSION

Unit	Description	Conversion	Remarks
Pressure			
Pa	Pascal	Standard unit	Pascal = Newton/ m^2
atm	Atmosphere (physical)	101,325 Pa	Pressure in gases
atm	Atmosphere (technical)	98,066.5 Pa	One atmosphere =1 kp/cm^2
bar	Bar	100,000 Pa	Pressure in gas and liquid
psi	Pounds per Square Inch	6,894.757293168 Pa	1 psi equivalent 14.5 bar
mbar	Millibar	100 Pa	Equivalent one hector pascal(hPa)
mmHg	Millimeter-mercury column	133.32 Pa	
Energy			
Unit	**Description**	**Conversion**	
J	Joule	Standard unit	
BTU	British Thermal Unit	1055.058138 J	
cal	calorie	4.186794846 J	
HPh	Horsepower hour	2684517.413 J	
Wh	Watt hour	3599.9982 J	
Area			
m^2	Square meter	Standard unit	
ha	Hectare	10,000 m^2	
ft^2	Square foot	0.0929 m^2	
km^2	Square kilometer	1,000,000 m^2	
mi^2	Square mile	2,589,988.11 m^2	
Volume			
l	Liter	Standard unit	
bl, bbl	Barrel	159 l	
gal	Gallon (UK)	4.55 l	
gal	Gallon (US)	3.7862 l	
pt	Pint	0.4733 l	
qt	Quart	0.9466 l	
Speed			

m/s	meters per second	Standard unit
km/h	kilometers per hour	0.278 m/s
mi/h	miles per hour	0.447 m/s
Power		
N	Newton	Standard unit
W	Watt	Standard unit
hp	horsepower	745.701 W
Length		
m	meter	Standard unit
ft	foot	0.3048 m
In	Inch	0.0254 m
mi	mile	1609.344 m
yd	yard	0.9144 m
Mass		
kg	kilogram	Standard unit
lb	pound	0.4536 kg
t	ton	1000 kg
oz	ounce	0.02834 kg
Temperature		
K	Kelvin	Standard unit
°C	Degree Celsius	K = °C+273.15
°F	Degree Fahrenheit	°F = 1.8×(K-273.15)+32
		$^{\circ}C = \frac{(^{\circ}F - 32)}{1.8}$
		°F = (°C×1.8)+32
Time		
s	second	Standard unit
m, min	minute	60 s
h	hour	3600 s
d	day	86400 s

FREQUENTLY USED STANDARDS OF CONCENTRATION

Measurement	Notation	Generic formula	Typical units
Mass percentage	wt% or w/w%	g solute x 100/ g solution	%
Mass-volume percentage	m/v%	g solute x100/ml solution	% though strictly % g/ml
Volume-volume percentage	vol% or v/v%	ml solute x 100/ ml solution	%
Molarity	M	moles solute/ liter solution	mol/l (or M or mol/ dm^3
Molinity	-	moles solute/ kg solution	mol/kg
Molality	m	moles solute/ kg solvent	mol/kg (or m)
Molar fraction	(chi)	moles solute/ moles solution	(decimal)
Formal	F	moles undissolved solute/liter solution	mol/l (or F)
Normality	N	gram equivalents/ liters solution	N
Parts per hundred	%(or pph)	Dekagrams solute/ kilograms solution	dg/kg
Parts per thousand	%(or ppt)	grams solute/ kilograms solution	g/kg
Parts per million	ppm	mg solute/kg solution	mg/kg
Parts per billion	ppb	µg solute/kg solution	µg/kg
Parts per trillion	ppt	ng solute/kg solution	ng/kg

❑❑❑